Aging
and Developmental Disability:
Current Research, Programming,
and Practice Implications

Aging and Developmental Disability: Current Research, Programming, and Practice Implications has been co-published simultaneously as *Physical & Occupational Therapy in Geriatrics,* Volume 18, Number 1 2000.

The *Physical & Occupational Therapy in Geriatrics* Monographic "Separates"

Below is a list of "separates," which in serials librarianship means a special issue simultaneously published as a special journal issue or double-issue *and* as a "separate" hardbound monograph. (This is a format which we also call a "DocuSerial.")

"Separates" are published because specialized libraries or professionals may wish to purchase a specific thematic issue by itself in a format which can be separately cataloged and shelved, as opposed to purchasing the journal on an on-going basis. Faculty members may also more easily consider a "separate" for classroom adoption.

"Separates" are carefully classified separately with the major book jobbers so that the journal tie-in can be noted on new book order slips to avoid duplicate purchasing.

You may wish to visit Haworth's website at . . .

http://www.HaworthPress.com

. . . to search our online catalog for complete tables of contents of these separates and related publications.

You may also call 1-800-HAWORTH (outside US/Canada: 607-722-5857), or Fax 1-800-895-0582 (outside US/Canada: 607-771-0012), or e-mail at:

getinfo@haworthpressinc.com

Aging and Developmental Disability: Current Research, Programming, and Practice Implications, edited by Joy Hammel, PhD, OTR/L, FAOTA, and Susan M. Nochajski, PhD, OTR/L (Vol. 18, No. 1, 2000). *Discusses the effectiveness of specific interventions targeted toward aging adults with developmental disabilities such as Down Syndrome, cerebral palsy, autism, and epilepsy.*

Teaching Students Geriatric Research, edited by Margaret A. Perkinson, PhD, and Kathryn L. Braun, DrPH (Vol. 17, No. 2, 2000). *"An excellent collection of well-written papers. . . . The presentation of each model is intriguing and will entice instructors to think about how they may enhance their approaches to working with graduate students in both classroom situations and as research assistants." (Karen A. Roberto, PhD, Professor and Director, Center for Gerontology, Virginia Polytechnic Institute and State University, Blacksburg, Virginia)*

Aging in Place: Designing, Adapting, and Enhancing the Home Environment, edited by Ellen D. Taira, OTR/L, MPH, and Jodi L. Carlson, MS, OTR/L (Vol. 16, No. 3/4, 1999). *This important book examines the current trends in adaptive home designs for older adults and explores innovative home designs and studies for creating environments that offer optimal living for aging adults.*

The Mentally Impaired Elderly: Strategies and Interventions to Maintain Function, edited by Ellen D. Taira, OTR/L, MPH (Vol. 9, No. 3/4, 1991). *"Caregivers will benefit from this book as it provides information on methods and strategies to deal with mentally impaired elderly patients." (Senior News)*

Aging in the Designed Environment, edited by Margaret A. Christenson, MPH, OTR (Vol. 8, No. 3/4, 1990). *"Presents the environment as the untapped treatment modality that can maximize a person's functional abilities when designed effectively . . . integrates theory with practice to provide a very coherent and stimulating book." (Canadian Journal of Occupational Therapy)*

Successful Models of Community Long Term Care Services for the Elderly, edited by Eloise H. P. Killeffer, EdM, and Ruth Bennett, PhD (Vol. 8, No. 1/2, 1990). *"Provides invaluable information to practitioners, educators, policymakers, and researchers concerned with meeting the myriad needs of the elderly." (Patricia A. Miller, MEd, OTR, FAOTA, Assistant Professor of Clinical Occupational Therapy and Public Health, Columbia University)*

Assessing the Driving Ability of the Elderly: A Preliminary Investigation, edited by Ellen D. Taira, OTR/L, MPH (Vol. 7, No. 1/2, 1989). *"'The' resource for older driver assessment. This new book provides a review of older driver literature, guidelines for practitioners who must assess older driver skills, and offers twenty-one screening instruments that test the visual, motor, and cognitive abilities of mature drivers." (Resources in Aging)*

Promoting Quality Long Term Care for Older Persons, edited by Ellen D. Taira, OTR/L, MPH (Vol. 6, No. 3/4, 1989). *Exciting programs in long term care–designed to better serve elderly persons with chronic diseases–are highlighted in this rich volume.*

Rehabilitation Interventions for the Institutionalized Elderly, edited by Ellen D. Taira, OTR/L, MPH (Vol. 6, No. 2, 1989). *"A sample of rehabilitation interventions which, combined in this volume, provide a holistic approach to gerontic services for those who are institutionalized." (Advances for Occupational Therapists)*

Community Programs for the Health Impaired Elderly, edited by Ellen D. Taira, OTR/L, MPH (Vol. 6, No. 1, 1989). *"This is an easy-to-read reference book occupational therapists can use to explore and develop techniques and programs to meet individual and community needs." (American Journal of Occupational Therapists)*

Community Programs for the Depressed Elderly: A Rehabilitation Approach, edited by Ellen D. Taira, OTR/L, MPH (Vol. 5, No. 1, 1987). *"A timely publication as recognition of the serious magnitude of depression amongst the elderly continues to grow." (Canadian Journal of Occupational Therapy)*

Therapeutic Interventions for the Person with Dementia, edited by Ellen D. Taira, OTR/L, MPH (Vol. 4, No. 3, 1986). *"Packed with useful information. The reader gains a better grasp of the patience, understanding, and flexibility needed to help these people. This is excellent reading for therapists and students and a valuable addition to the library of anyone working with the elderly." (American Journal of Occupational Therapy)*

Handbook of Innovative Programs for the Impaired Elderly, edited by Eloise H. P. Killeffer, EdM, Ruth Bennett, PhD, and Gerta Gruen, MPH (Vol. 3, No. 3, 1985). *"A handy source of ideas for promoting maintenance of physical abilities, restoring physical and mental abilities, and linking residents with organizations and services in the surrounding community and opening the long-term care facility to the community." (Canadian Journal of Occupational Therapy)*

A Handbook of Assistive Devices for the Handicapped Elderly: New Help for Independent Living, by Joseph M. Breuer, MA, RPT (Vol. 1, No. 2, 1982). *"Practical advice is coupled with a significant theoretical background and valuable experience." (Journal of the American Geriatrics Society)*

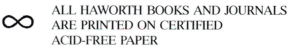

Aging
and Developmental Disability:
Current Research,
Programming,
and Practice Implications

Joy Hammel, PhD, OTR/L, FAOTA
Susan M. Nochajski, PhD, OTR/L
Editors

Aging and Developmental Disability: Current Research, Programming, and Practice Implications has been co-published simultaneously as *Physical & Occupational Therapy in Geriatrics*, Volume 18, Number 1 2000.

The Haworth Press, Inc.
New York • London • Oxford

Aging and Developmental Disability: Current Research, Programming, and Practice Implications has been co-published simultaneously as *Physical & Occupational Therapy in Geriatrics,* Volume 18, Number 1 2000.

The Haworth Press, Inc., 10 Alice Street, Binghamton, NY 13904-1580 USA

Cover design by Thomas J. Mayshock Jr.

Library of Congress Cataloging-in-Publication Data

Aging and developmental disability: current research, programming, and practice implications / Joy Hammel, Susan M. Nochajski, editors.
     p. cm.
     "Has been co-published simultaneously as Physical & occupational therapy in geriatrics, volume 18, number 1, 2000."
     Includes bibliographical references and index.
     ISBN 0-7890-1039-9 (alk. paper) – ISBN 0-7890-1040-2 (alk. paper)
     1. Developmentally disabled aged. 2. Developmentally disabled aged–Services for. 3. Physical therapy for the aged. I. Hammel, Joy. II. Nochajski, Susan M. III. Physical & occupational therapy in geriatrics.
HV3009.5.A35 A355 2001
362.1'968–dc21

00-049890

Indexing, Abstracting & Website/Internet Coverage

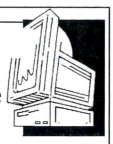

This section provides you with a list of major indexing & abstracting services. That is to say, each service began covering this periodical during the year noted in the right column. Most Websites which are listed below have indicated that they will either post, disseminate, compile, archive, cite or alert their own Website users with research-based content from this work. (This list is as current as the copyright date of this publication.)

(continued)

(continued)

Special Bibliographic Notes related to special journal issues
(separates) and indexing/abstracting:

- indexing/abstracting services in this list will also cover material in any "separate" that is co-published simultaneously with Haworth's special thematic journal issue or DocuSerial. Indexing/abstracting usually covers material at the article/chapter level.
- monographic co-editions are intended for either non-subscribers or libraries which intend to purchase a second copy for their circulating collections.
- monographic co-editions are reported to all jobbers/wholesalers/approval plans. The source journal is listed as the "series" to assist the prevention of duplicate purchasing in the same manner utilized for books-in-series.
- to facilitate user/access services all indexing/abstracting services are encouraged to utilize the co-indexing entry note indicated at the bottom of the first page of each article/chapter/contribution.
- this is intended to assist a library user of any reference tool (whether print, electronic, online, or CD-ROM) to locate the monographic version if the library has purchased this version but not a subscription to the source journal.
- individual articles/chapters in any Haworth publication are also available through the Haworth Document Delivery Service (HDDS).

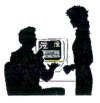

Aging and Developmental Disability: Current Research, Programming, and Practice Implications

CONTENTS

ABOUT THE EDITORS

Joy Hammel, PhD, OTR/L, FAOTA, is Assistant Professor in the Departments of Occupational Therapy and Disability and Human Development, and on the faculty of the Joint Doctoral Program in Disability Studies at the University of Illinois at Chicago. She received her PhD in Educational Psychology from the University of California, Berkeley, and her BS in Occupational Therapy from the University of Wisconsin, Madison. Dr. Hammel has worked as an OTR for over 13 years, served as past Chair of the American Occupational Therapy Special Interest Section, and is currently Principal Investigator on several federal research grants. Her research focuses on the supports and barriers to community living experienced by disabled people and older adults, including the long term use, outcomes, and funding of assistive technology and environmental interventions.

Susan M. Nochajski, PhD, OTR/L, is Assistant Professor in the Department of Occupational Therapy at the University at Buffalo, The State University of New York. Dr. Nochajski has BS and MS degrees in Occupational Therapy and a PhD in Special Education from the University at Buffalo. She has over twenty years of clinical experience in occupational therapy working primarily with persons of all ages with developmental disabilities. Dr. Nochajski's current research interests involve the use and functional impact of assistive technology by persons with disabilities, particularly by persons with intellectual disabilities as they age and by students with disabilities as they transition from secondary education to adult settings.

Introduction:
Aging and Developmental Disability: Current Research, Programming, and Practice Implications

Joy Hammel, PhD, OTR/L, FAOTA
Susan M. Nochajski, PhD, OTR/L

The concepts of aging in place, healthy aging, and life course planning have become central themes within policy and funding agencies and programming initiatives; they also represent emerging areas of practice as therapists expand into health and wellness programming across the lifespan within community and long term care settings. Aging research has increasingly focused on the experiences of people with long term disabilities, such as developmental disabilities, as they age. This volume on Developmental Disability and Aging explores

Joy Hammel is Assistant Professor, Occupational Therapy Department, University of Illinois at Chicago, 1919 West Taylor Street, Room 311, Chicago, IL 60612 (E-mail: hammel@uic.edu). Susan M. Nochajski is Assistant Professor, Occupational Therapy Department, State University of New York, 515 Kimball Tower, Buffalo, NY 14214 (E-mail: nochajsk@acsu.buffalo.edu).

Preparation of this article was supported in part by funding from the Rehabilitation Research and Training Center on Aging with Mental Retardation, University of Illinois at Chicago, through the U.S. Department of Education, National Institute on Disability and Rehabilitation Research, Grant number H133B980046. The opinions contained in this publication are those of the grantee and do not necessarily reflect those of the U.S. Department of Education.

[Haworth co-indexing entry note]: "Introduction: *Aging and Developmental Disability: Current Research, Programming, and Practice Implications*." Hammel, Joy, and Susan M. Nochajski. Co-published simultaneously in *Physical & Occupational Therapy in Geriatrics* (The Haworth Press, Inc.) Vol. 18, No. 1, 2000, pp. 1-4; and: *Aging and Developmental Disability: Current Research, Programming, and Practice Implications* (ed: Joy Hammel, and Susan M. Nochajski) The Haworth Press, Inc., 2000, pp. 1-4. Single or multiple copies of this article are available for a fee from The Haworth Document Delivery Service [1-800-342-9678, 9:00 a.m. - 5:00 p.m. (EST). E-mail address: getinfo@haworthpressinc.com].

research findings and practice implications regarding normative and disability-related aging experiences and issues, effectiveness of specific interventions targeted toward aging adults with developmental disabilities and their caregivers, and implications for practice and future research in this area.

According to the Developmental Disabilities Assistance and Bill of Rights Act (2000) (currently under reauthorization consideration), developmental disability is defined as a "severe, chronic disability of an individual that is attributable to a mental or physical impairment or combination of mental and physical impairments; is manifested before the individual attains age 22; is likely to continue indefinitely; and results in substantial functional limitations in 3 or more of the following areas of major life activity: self-care, receptive and expressive language, learning, mobility, self-direction, capacity for independent living, and economic self-sufficiency." Disabilities such as mental retardation, Down Syndrome, cerebral palsy, autism and epilepsy would be considered developmental disabilities. Many individuals experience a combination of conditions that may result in motor, sensory, cognitive, intellectual, and/or psychosocial impairments. This volume primarily will focus upon people with intellectual disabilities, alone or in combination with other impairments.

According to the reauthorization proposal, there are between 3,200,000 and 4,500,000 individuals with developmental disabilities in the United States as of 1999, comprising between 1.2 and 1.65 percent of the United States population (Developmental Disabilities Act, 2000). There are an estimated 526,000 people over age 60 with mental retardation and other developmental disabilities; this number is predicted to double by the year 2030 (Heller & Factor, 1998). The majority of people with developmental disabilities live with families or in community-based group homes, although a significant number reside in multi-bed, long term care settings such as Intermediate Care Facilities, nursing homes and institutions. Over 479,000 adults with developmental disabilities are living at home with parents who are 60 years old or older and who serve as the primary caregivers (Developmental Disabilities Act, 2000). These numbers demonstrate an increasing population of people with developmental disabilities, and their caregivers, who are or will be aging in place in a range of settings with diverse medical, functional, independent living, and social issues and needs.

The first two articles in this volume describe this population of aging adults with developmental disabilities. Nochajski summarizes normative and disability-related aging processes within the general older adult population, and contrasts these with current findings regarding aging with life long developmental disabilities. Recent research points to potentially earlier and increased occurrence of select normative aging and disability-related processes among adults with developmental disabilities. These changes may or may not result in functional limitations and decreased community participation, depending on early identification and targeted intervention, programming, and education to address, prevent or delay such outcomes.

Gill and Brown focus upon recognizing and identifying the specific needs of women with intellectual disabilities as they age. As shown in the article, women with disabilities face unique health and communication issues that closely interact with participation in everyday activities, community living, and social relationships. Therapists need to closely listen to these needs and actively collaborate with women when creating individualized health and wellness plans and community-based programs.

The next three articles focus on interventions and programming for persons with developmental disabilities who are aging, and their caregivers and important others in their lives. Using the International Classification of Functioning (ICIDH-2) (WHO, 2000) as an organizing framework, Hammel discusses the available range and impact of assistive technology and environmental interventions for aging adults with developmental disabilities, and their caregivers, across impairment, activity, participation, and environmental levels. Assessment and intervention implications for therapists in their roles as interface specialists and community consultants are offered.

Heller presents a literature review of life course planning programs and research focused upon enabling people with developmental disabilities, and important others, to make choices and informed decisions about living situation, estate planning, physical assistance, social support, and activity programming as they age. This article focuses on issues related to self-advocacy and empowerment as critical tools for community living and later-life planning.

Campbell and Herge discuss the challenges to aging in place that are experienced by older adults with developmental disabilities, their families and the service community. The article describes the role of occupational and physical therapists in assisting the older adult to age in place in the community.

Finally, information resources on aging and developmental disabilities policy, legislation, programming, product vendors and reviews, and research findings are provided at the end of this volume. Many of the resources are located on the World Wide Web, with links to other sites, databases and organizations. Therapists can play a critical role as educators in linking consumers and important others to these resources so they can stay informed and assume self-advocacy roles related to their own health and wellness.

REFERENCES

Developmental Disabilities Assistance and Bill of Rights Act of 1999 (reauthorization proposal dated 1/29/2000). American Association of University Affiliated Programs. Website: <http://www.aauap.org/legisaff/main.html>.
Heller, T., & Factor, A. (1998). Research advances and research directions on aging with mental retardation. Chicago, IL: Aging and MR RRTC Clearinghouse, UIC.
WHO (2000). *ICIDH-2: International Classification of Functioning and Disability.* Website address: <http://www.who.int/icidh/index.htm> (1/20/2000). Geneva: World Health Organization.

The Impact of Age-Related Changes on the Functioning of Older Adults with Developmental Disabilities

Susan M. Nochajski, PhD, OTR/L

SUMMARY. This paper discusses age-related changes that have an impact on functional abilities and societal participation of older adults with mental retardation. A description of changes that affect all older individuals is presented as well as the additional impact these changes may have on older persons with developmental disabilities. Information on age-related changes unique to persons with Down Syndrome and cerebral palsy are also presented. The role of occupational and physical therapists in helping to maintain the functional abilities of aging persons with developmental disabilities is discussed. *[Article copies available for a fee from The Haworth Document Delivery Service: 1-800-342-9678. E-mail address: <getinfo@haworthpressinc.com> Website: <http://www.HaworthPress.com>]*

KEYWORDS. Aging, developmental disabilities, functional abilities

INTRODUCTION

In our society, we typically think of 65 as the beginning of late adulthood. The group of individuals over 65 years, and more specifically, those over 85, is the most rapidly growing age group in the

Susan M. Nochajski is Assistant Professor, Department of Occupational Therapy, State University of New York at Buffalo, 515 Kimball Tower, Buffalo, NY 14214 (E-mail: nochajsk@acsu.buffalo.edu).

[Haworth co-indexing entry note]: "The Impact of Age-Related Changes on the Functioning of Older Adults with Developmental Disabilities." Nochajski, Susan M. Co-published simultaneously in *Physical & Occupational Therapy in Geriatrics* (The Haworth Press, Inc.) Vol. 18, No. 1, 2000, pp. 5-21; and: *Aging and Developmental Disability: Current Research, Programming, and Practice Implications* (ed: Joy Hammel, and Susan M. Nochajski) The Haworth Press, Inc., 2000, pp. 5-21. Single or multiple copies of this article are available for a fee from The Haworth Document Delivery Service [1-800-342-9678, 9:00 a.m. - 5:00 p.m. (EST). E-mail address: getinfo@haworthpressinc.com].

5

United States (Herr & Weber, 1999). According to the U.S. Senate Special Committee on Aging (1991), the percentage of the U.S. population over the age of 65 has grown from 8% in 1950, to 12% in 1990 and is expected to increase to over 14% by 2000. This also includes persons with developmental disabilities; approximately 12% of the persons with developmental disabilities are over the age of 65. This figure is similar to the percentage of individuals without disabilities in the same age group (Connolly, 1998).

Concurrent with a growth in the number of persons over 65, the life expectancy of these individuals is also increasing. The current mean age at death for persons with and without disabilities is approximately 70 years (Braddock, 1999; Herr & Weber, 1999). Individuals with Down Syndrome currently have a life expectancy of 60-64 years and people with other types of developmental disabilities have a life expectancy of 70-74 years (Strauss and Eyman, 1996). This is a dramatic contrast from 1930 when the life expectancy for persons with mental retardation was approximately 20 years (Carter & Jancar, 1983 cited in Herr & Weber, 1999) and that of a person with Down Syndrome was only 9 years (Penrose, 1949 cited in Herr & Weber, 1999).

Aging is a developmental process that starts at birth and involves gradual changes in body structures and systems. Although we all experience age-related changes, not everyone experiences changes at the same rate and these changes do not have the same impact on everyone. When they occur, however, they can have an impact on an individual's functional performance and societal participation. Dysfunction occurs as the result of several processes including chronic conditions associated with developmental disability, the severity of the disability, age-related changes, and other disease processes. Whether or not a person experiences limits on his or her functional abilities and social participation is affected by heredity, life style, overall health, and the environment.

This article addresses a description of, and select research findings, related to the impairment level of disability as described in the International Classification of Functioning (WHO, 2000). Topics presented in this article include:

- age-related changes typically found in the general population;
- the impact these changes may have on aging adults with developmental disabilities;

- age-related changes unique to persons with Down Syndrome and cerebral palsy;
- the role of occupational and physical therapists in helping to maintain an individual's functional abilities.

PHYSICAL CHANGES ASSOCIATED WITH AGING AND THEIR IMPACT ON FUNCTION

Biological aging produces changes that effect all body organs and · systems. It is important to remember that these are interrelated and changes in one system will have an effect on other systems. Age-related changes are discussed here as separate systems only for clarity in presentation.

Nervous System

As a person ages, changes occur in the central nervous system. Within the brain, there is: (a) diminished blood flow; (b) a gradual loss of neurons; (c) a decreased number of cells; (d) a decrease in the number of synaptic interconnections; (e) increased synaptic delay; and (f) decreases in neurotransmitter activity (Machemer & Overeynder, 1993; Mann & Hurren, 1994; Miller, 1992). As a result of these changes in the central nervous system, as well as the peripheral nervous system, older persons may experience problems with their ability to receive, process and respond to stimuli (Miller, 1992). For example, an older person may experience a decreased reaction time or a decreased speed of recall. However, changes in cognitive functioning, such as a decline in intelligence or a major loss of memory are not typical age-related nervous system changes.

Sensory Systems

Age-related changes occur in all sensory systems–visual, auditory, tactile, proprioceptive, gustatory and olfactory, but those related to vision and hearing may occur earlier in persons with developmental disabilities and have a greater impact on function than in the general population (Machemer and Overeynder, 1993).

Vision: Close to 95% of people over the age of 65 wear glasses (Connolly, 1998). With increasing age, structural changes in the eye affect vision and impact on functional abilities (Christenson, 1990).

Structural changes include: (a) increased lens size and density; (b) a flattening and decrease in elasticity of the lens; (c) increased hardening and rigidity of the iris; (d) smaller pupil size due to rigidity of the iris; and (e) degeneration of neurons in the visual cortex (Miller, 1992).

Presbyopia is one of the earliest conditions resulting from structural changes in the eye. As the lens ages, old cells are not shed, but "build up" leading to a yellowing of the lens. This yellowing of the lens makes it more difficult for an individual to distinguish between blue-green and yellow-white colors. Additionally, the yellowing of the lens decreases clarity and increases glare (Miller, 1992). The decrease in pupil size results in an increased sensitivity to glare and difficulty with adaptation to the dark. Other structural changes within the eye result in altered depth perception, a narrowing of the visual field, changes in color vision, and slower processing of visual information (Mann & Hurren, 1994; Miller, 1992). Disease processes, such as the development of cataracts and glaucoma, have an effect on an individual's visual abilities, but these are not "normal" age-related changes (Miller, 1992).

Hearing: It has been reported that 23% of persons between the ages of 65 and 74 experience a significant hearing loss; increasing to 34% between 75 and 84 and to 51% over the age of 85. Degenerative changes affect all components of the ear and the entire auditory nerve pathway resulting in a condition known as presbycusis. Presbycusis is a sensorineural hearing loss that interferes with the person's ability to hear high pitched sounds. When high pitched sounds are filtered out, words become distorted and sentences incoherent, making conversations difficult (Miller, 1992). Problems due to hearing loss are often erroneously viewed by others as senility.

Degeneration of the auditory nerve and a decreased blood supply to neurosensory receptors can lead to a condition known as tinnitus, more commonly known as "ringing in the ears." Older adults with tinnitus have difficulty hearing conversations, door bells and sirens (Mann & Hurren, 1994).

Smell/Taste: Research suggests that as persons become older, there is a decreased sensitivity in both olfactory and gustatory receptors. Degenerative changes in the olfactory system start around the age of 30 and the sense of smell is almost completely diminished by the time a person reaches 80. These changes often make food unappealing and can lead to a decrease in appetite that will compromise the person's nutritional status (Connolly, 1998). The loss of smell also presents health and safety concerns for older individuals. For example, a person may become ill if he or she is unable to detect the smell of spoiled food before it is eaten. The loss of smell also presents safety concerns if the individual can not smell a gas leak or food burning.

Somatosensory: A decreased sensitivity in touch receptors and slowing of nerve impulse transmissions causes a decreased response to tactile stimuli. This can result in decreased sensitivity to touch, pain, pressure, and temperature extremes (Mann & Hurren, 1994).

Impact of Sensory and Nervous System Changes: Diminishing sensory abilities and decreased activity in the nervous system lead to problems for older adults in many areas of functioning that are important for their well-being, safety, and quality of life. For example, age-related changes in the nervous system that result in a decline in the speed of information processing may decrease the individual's ability to adapt to, and use new information, in reasoning or problem solving. Visual changes may affect a person's ability to drive a vehicle, go up and down stairs, or read; hearing deficits may lead to social isolation. The decreased sensitivity to taste and smell can affect appetite and nutritional intake. These changes may effect the functioning of all persons as they age. However, individuals with developmental disabilities, because of their judgement or prior life experiences, may be at an increased risk for loss of function due to these changes.

Musculoskeletal System

Skeletal Components: Osteoarthritis is a chronic condition that is perhaps the most universally acknowledged indicator of aging. This condition, caused by deterioration of articular cartilage and the reformation of new bone at the joint surfaces, occurs in approximately 75% of the population by age 75 and in over 90% by the age of 80. Although it is typically not found in individuals younger than 40, osteoarthritis reportedly occurs at younger ages in persons with developmental disabilities (Connolly, 1998). General symptoms of osteoarthritis include stiffness, pain and discomfort, limited range of motion and joint hypertrophy; characteristics of more severe forms may include contractures, joint deformity, posture changes, and fine and gross motor impairments (Miller, 1992).

Osteoporosis, the increased porosity or "softening" of the bone structure, is another chronic condition that occurs in older adults that is generally characterized by low bone mass density and deterioration of bone tissue (Center, Beange, & McElduff, 1998). Although bone growth stops in early adulthood, bone remodeling continues throughout adulthood. In older adults, the "softening" of bone affects the remodeling process causing a decrease in density that makes a person susceptible to fractures (Miller, 1992).

Muscular Components: As a person ages, changes occur in skeletal, cardiac and smooth muscles including: (a) a decreased number or motor neurons; (b) a loss of muscle mass; (c) deterioration of and decrease in the number of muscle fibers; and (d) deterioration of the muscle cell membranes (Miller, 1992). There is a gradual diminishing of muscle strength and endurance, a slower speed of muscle contraction and problems with both fine and gross motor coordination (Machemer and Overeynder, 1993; Miller, 1992). Muscle strength decreases from 25 to 43%, depending on the individual's activity level. A decline in the strength of the anti-gravity muscles, such as the hip flexors, quadriceps, and triceps is more apt to occur when an individual is inactive (Connolly, 1998).

Impact of Musculoskeletal Changes: One of the most significant consequences of age-related changes in the musculoskeletal system is the impact of the combination of skeletal, muscular, and neurological changes on gait and balance. Osteoporosis and other age-related changes are responsible for a height loss of approximately 2 to 4 cm per decade of adult life (Connolly, 1998). The calcification of cartilage in the thoracic wall and muscle atrophy contribute toward the development of a kyphotic or "stooped" posture, with a slight forward flexion of the head and neck and flexion of the knees and hips. When an individual is inactive and remains in one position, particularly sitting, for extended periods of time, there is tendency for the flexor muscles in the body to shorten resulting in a "stooped" posture (Connolly, 1998). This posture changes the center of gravity and impedes a person's ability to maintain balance (Miller, 1992). Poor balance often leads to falls which have very serious consequences for persons with osteoporosis. Balance is also affected by age-related changes in proprioceptive abilities and the vestibular system in the inner ear.

As a result of musculoskeletal changes, older adults may develop alternate gait patterns. Women may develop a "waddling" gait, with a narrower base of support for walking and standing. Due to decreased muscular control, there is also a tendency for women to develop bow-legged type postures that alter the angle of the hips and affect the lower extremities. These changes predispose women to both falls and fractures. On the other hand, the gait of older men becomes wider and is characterized by a flexed position of the head and trunk, decreased arm swing, a shorter stride, and the feet barely raised from the surface (Miller, 1992). As a result of the "waddling" gait in women and the "shuffling" gait in men, both groups spend more time in the support rather than swing phase of gait and have a slower speed of walking.

Other Systems

Age-related changes in the nervous, sensory and musculoskeletal systems are perhaps the most familiar to therapists and may be viewed, from a therapy perspective, as having a significant impact on an individual's functional abilities. However, age-related changes occur in other systems including the cardiovascular, respiratory, gastrointestinal, urinary, and integumentary systems. Herge and Campbell (1998) and Mann and Hurren (1994) have discussed the age-related changes and concerns in these systems that are most relevant to functional status. This information is briefly summarized below.

Cardiovascular System: Whether structural and physiological changes within the heart and cardiovascular system are due to age-related changes or lifestyle choices has been widely debated. Whatever the etiology, as individuals age, they often experience up to a 40% decrease in cardiac output (Mann & Hurren, 1994). There is also increased peripheral resistance to arterial blood flow resulting in compensatory blood pressure increases and a decreased elasticity in cardiac valves and blood vessels. Due to decreased sensitivity in the baroreceptors, nerve ending that are stimulated by changes in pressure, older adults may also experience orthostatic hypotension, that is, altered blood pressure regulation with position change (i.e., feeling dizzy when they get out of bed too quickly) (Herge & Campbell, 1998; Mann & Hurren, 1994). As a result of these changes, older adults may experience decreased endurance and a diminished cardiovascular response to high stress or high demand situations that will require them to pace activities and conserve energy.

Respiratory System: With increasing age, there are skeletal changes, such as an increase in the antero-posterior chest diameter, and muscular changes, such as a general weakening of the respiratory muscles. These changes lead to a decreased vital capacity and the amount of oxygen available for gas exchange. There is also a decrease in the number of alveoli in the lungs and a thickening of the membranes involved in gas exchange which can lead to shortness of breath and fatigue (Mann & Hurren, 1994).

Gastrointestinal System: Common age-related occurrences in this system include changes in the teeth, gingivae and alveolar ridge that result in a decreased ability to chew, dry mouth, or ill-fitting dentures. As a person ages, he or she also experiences decreases in saliva production and diminished esophageal peristalsis that can cause difficulty with swallowing. There is also inadequate relaxation of the lower esophagus which decreases gastric emptying and can lead to heartburn or a hiatal hernia (Herge & Campbell, 1998). Decreased peristalsis throughout the gastrointestinal system, which can lead to chronic constipation, is also common. Perhaps the most significant change in the gastrointestinal system is a decrease in the absorptive area in the small intestine. With increased age, the villi become fewer in number and there is less surface area to absorb nutrients resulting in an increased likelihood of malnutrition (Mann & Hurren, 1994).

Urinary System: A decrease in the number of nephrons and overall renal blood flow can lead to a decreased filtration rate of the kidney, reduced efficiency in removing wastes from the body, and diminish the absorption of some types of medication. The electrolyte balance is easily disrupted by losses of fluid through diarrhea, vomiting, or lack of fluid intake; this imbalance can lead to serious renal insufficiency. There is also a decrease in bladder muscle tone and overall bladder capacity resulting in changes in urinary frequency and urgency (Mann & Hurren, 1994).

Integumentary System: As a person ages, the sweat glands diminish in number, size and function resulting in an inability to regulate heat and maintain body temperatures in hot weather conditions. There is also a thinning of the skin and an increased fragility of the blood vessels under the surface of the skin that makes older adults susceptible to bruising (Mann & Hurren, 1994).

Impact of Changes in Other Systems: Age-related changes in these systems, although not frequently considered, have a substantial impact on the functional activity and societal participation of older adults. Decreased endurance and stamina due to cardiovascular and respiratory changes may force an individual to limit his or her activities. Due to changes within the urinary system, such as increased frequency and urgency in voiding, an individual may limit social activities, particularly if accessible rest rooms are not conveniently located. Conversely, a person may participate in social activities but limit his or her amount of fluid intake to avoid needing to use the restroom; this can compromise health status.

AGING WITH A DEVELOPMENTAL DISABILITY

Persons with mental retardation and other developmental disabilities experience the same age-related changes that occur in individuals without disabilities with the same medical and mental health problems that occur in the general population (Hotaling, 1998). The majority of age-related changes previously described occur similarly in the general population and among persons with developmental disabilities (Machemer and Overeynder, 1993). However, as Connolly (1998) suggests, the aging process may start earlier in persons with mental retardation and other developmental disabilities, perhaps as early as age 35. Lubin and Kiley (1985) have suggested that age-related changes are likely to occur, not only at an earlier age, but also at a faster rate among persons with developmental disabilities, particularly those with Down Syndrome, than in the general population. Therefore, whether or not chronological age is an appropriate measure when looking at aging issues effecting persons with developmental disabilities remains inconclusive.

The onset and impact of age-related changes are influenced by the severity of the person's existing disabilities and are likely to have a more significant effect if the person has more than one defined developmental disability. Using retrospective data, Brzezniak (1998) evaluated the aging process of 103 persons with developmental disabilities with respect to their ability to ambulate independently. Over a 10 year period, 11.8% of the sample with only one disability lost their ability to ambulate independently; this increased to 16% if two disabilities were present. The greatest decrease in functional ambulation occurred if an individual had three or more conditions; 62.9% of this group lost their independent ambulation skills. The most significant decline occurred in individuals with a combination of mental retardation, cerebral palsy, and epilepsy.

Burdett (1998) reports there were not significant differences in health status or the number of medical conditions between a matched group of older persons with and without developmental disabilities.

Findings such as these help to explain similarities in life expectancy between the two groups. However, as might be expected, individuals with health and medical conditions that pre-date the onset of age-related changes have a shorter life expectancy. Research has shown that persons with profound mental retardation were more apt to have higher mortality rates associated with respiratory disease than were persons functioning at other levels (Jenkins, Hildreth, & Hildreth, 1993). Additionally, persons who have severe motor impairments or require tube feeding also have a lower life expectancy (Jenkins, Hildreth, & Hildreth, 1993).

Persons with developmental disabilities, particularly those with cerebral palsy or Down Syndrome, were found to be more likely to develop osteoporosis at an earlier age than persons in the general population (Center et al., 1998). Immobility and a deficiency in vitamin K were found to be contributing factors to the development of osteoporosis (Wagemans, Fiolet, van der Linden, & Menheere, 1998). Although osteoporosis predisposes a person to fractures, there are also reports of a high incidence of fractures in persons with epilepsy (Lohiya, Lohiya, & Tan-Figuerroa, 1999). Prolonged use of anti-epileptic drugs may produce osteomalacia, a condition that predisposes a person to fractures.

Individuals with developmental disabilities, as do all individuals, experience age-related changes that impact on their functional abilities and interpersonal interactions. Although conditions associated with a developmental disability may increase the functional impact of certain age-related changes, it cannot be assumed functional changes occur merely as a result of a chronic condition associated with the developmental disability.

Aging with Down Syndrome

Down Syndrome (DS), caused by the presence of extra material on chromosome 21, is one of the most common genetic disorders that results in varying levels of severity of mental retardation. Over the past two decades, research has been instrumental in developing an understanding of the medical needs of persons with DS resulting in a notable increase in life expectancy (Fenderson, 1998).

Physical Concerns: Older adults with DS have many unique medical needs and concerns (Burt et al., 1995). There is a higher prevalence of epilepsy, an increased susceptibility to infection, and hypothyroidism. Functional consequences of hypothyroidism include lethargy, fatigue, diminished participation in activities of daily living, confusion, and depression (Fenderson, 1998). Zigman, Silverman, and Wisniewski (1996) report that congenital heart malformations, such as the Tetraology of Fallot, are estimated to be present in 35% to 60% of the individuals with DS. Although corrective surgery is now performed during childhood, many older adults with DS have uncorrected abnormalities that may lead to cardiac problems. There is a greater prevalence of mitral valve prolapse in older adults with DS than in the general population (Fenderson, 1998). Additionally, the medical needs of older persons with DS who have had corrective surgery are not known (Fenderson, 1998).

There is a high incidence of visual and auditory problems in persons with DS that appear to become more severe with age. Strabismus, nystagmus, refractive errors of the lens and cataracts are visual problems frequently encountered by persons with DS. Fenderson (1998) notes that the incidence of cataracts has been reported to be as high as 46% of the population. The excessive accumulation and impaction of ear wax leads to auditory problems. The chronic nature of these conditions is a major contributing factor to the sensorineural hearing loss that frequently occurs in adults with DS.

There are many abnormalities in the musculoskeletal systems of individuals with DS. Hypotonia is a distinguishing feature of DS that occurs in 88% to 98% of the population. Ligamentous laxity, along with hypotonia, leads to hyperflexibility of the joints. This in turn causes orthopedic and motor problems for persons with DS, the most significant being atlantoaxial (AA) instability (Fenderson, 1998). AA instability is described below.

The atlas and axis of the cervical spine meet with the occiput at the base of the neck and are stabilized with connections between bone, muscle, and ligaments. The transverse ligament prevents excessive motion of the atlas anteriorly and the axis posteriorly. However, laxity of the transverse ligament in persons with DS leads to AA instability. While usually asymptomatic, AA dislocation or subluxation can lead to compression of the spinal cord, quadriplegia, and possible death (Fenderson, 1998).

Alzheimer's Disease and DS: It has been well documented that adults with DS have a greater likelihood of developing Alzheimer's disease or dementia-like symptoms than the general population (Burt et al., 1995) and numerous studies have investigated the relationship between these two conditions (Silverman, Zigman, Kim, Krinsky-

McHale, and Wisniewski, 1998). Fenderson (1998) cites several studies suggesting that results from postmortem autopsies indicate that the majority of adults with DS will develop the neurofibrillary tangles and neuritic plaques characteristic of Alzheimer's disease by the time they reach 40 years of age. However, recent research has found that despite the presence of neurologic changes characteristic of Alzheimer's disease, many adults with DS do not have impairment of functional skills, regress with age, or demonstrate changes in behavior or personality (Zigman et al., 1996). Research is needed that provides more information about the normal aging process in persons with DS before the relationship between Alzheimer's disease and DS can be fully ascertained (Baird & Sadovnick, 1988).

Summary: While there is an abundance of literature describing the physical and cognitive age-related changes that are specific to persons with DS, there is scant research that explores the impact of these changes on functional activity, such as activities of daily living or instrumental activities of daily living. This is an area that needs to be further investigated.

Aging with Cerebral Palsy

There are currently over 400,000 adults with cerebral palsy in the United States and the number is growing due to advances in medicine and rehabilitation and the resultant increase in life-expectancy (Murphy, Molnar, & Lankasky, 1995). However, Overeynder and Turk (1998) indicate that little empirical research exists as to whether persons with cerebral palsy age in ways similar or different to the general population. Anecdotal information provided by persons with cerebral palsy reported unanticipated problems with fatigue, pain, increased spasticity, deconditioning, balance and oral motor problems. These problems impact on their functional abilities and can affect their ability to continue life roles. Research needs to be conducted to investigate whether these problems are typical for the majority of persons with cerebral palsy, whether these problems are preventable, and whether decreased functional abilities occur at an earlier age than in the general population.

Empirical information, albeit scant, does appear in the literature. In a study by Murphy et al. (1995), musculoskeletal problems were found to be prevalent in a group of persons with cerebral palsy (n = 106) and these problems initially occurred at a relatively young age. Fifty-four percent of the participants under the age of 50 experienced cervical pain, 44% experienced back pain and 27% reported pain in weight bearing joints. In participants between the ages of 50 and 74, the percentages of those participants reporting pain increased considerably. Twenty-one percent of the participants under the age of 50 reported muscle pain and spasms. This problem was not reported in the 50 to 74 year age group, but 84% of the older participants reported lower extremity contractures and 29% reported contractures in the upper extremities. The apparent lack of medical or therapeutic intervention is an area of concern for these individuals.

It appears that the impact of age-related changes on individuals with cerebral palsy is dependent on the extent and severity of their life-long disability; this is another area which warrants further investigation.

IMPLICATIONS FOR OCCUPATIONAL AND PHYSICAL THERAPISTS

Occupational and physical therapists and other health care and service providers need to have knowledge of the physical changes that occur as a person ages (Herge & Campbell, 1998). This article summarizes these physical changes. However, knowledge of changes that occur at the impairment level of disability classification is not enough. Therapists need to consider the impact of these physical changes on a person's daily roles and activities.

Therapists need to be able to assess these changes and their impact on functional activities, develop appropriate interventions, and share this information with the person with the developmental disability and his or her care providers. Hotaling (1998) suggests that therapists need to use a holistic and multi-dimensional perspective to meet the wide-ranging needs of older adults with developmental disabilities. This perspective focuses on functional activities and should include a variety of components including therapeutic activities, education for service and care providers, environmental modifications, temporal modifications and the use of adaptive equipment. Hammel (2000), in another article in this volume, provides information on assistive technology and environmental modifications as interventions that can have a positive impact on an individual's functioning at the activity, participation, and societal levels.

Perhaps one of the most important roles for therapists and other service providers is the promotion of wellness and a healthy lifestyle for older persons with developmental disabilities. Research by Clark et al. (1997) suggests that preventative health programs focusing on activity lessen the health risks of older adulthood. Older adults are able to minimize the effects of age-related changes, such as muscle tone, joint flexibility and physical stamina and endurance through a healthy lifestyle that includes regular exercise (Miller, 1992).

This article primarily addresses the physical aspects of aging. However, in using a holistic approach, such as that advocated by Hotaling (1998), occupational and physical therapists need to be cognizant of the psychosocial and mental health issues individuals face as they age. Moss (1999) notes that the study of mental health problems in older persons with developmental disabilities is relatively new. However, it can be assumed that the trends for age-related mental illnesses among people with and without developmental disabilities is similar, with depression and anxiety being the most prevalent disorders. Physical factors, such as the association between paranoid psychoses and temporal lobe epilepsy and severe visual and hearing impairments, play a role in the development of mental illness (Moss, 1999). However, more commonly, depression and anxiety are related to facing and coping with major life changes and losses that accompany aging (Ludlow, 1999). The reader is referred to Day and Jancar (1994) for further information in this area.

CONCLUSION

During the past two decades, aging in persons with developmental disabilities, particularly intellectual disabilities, has become a central issue for researchers and service providers (Hogg, 1997). Although the life expectancy for persons with developmental disabilities is increasing, longevity without quality of life is problematic. Janicki, Dalton, Henderson, and Davidson (1999) suggest that there is a need for research to evaluate the factors that contribute to successful aging by persons with developmental disabilities. Longitudinal studies are also needed to determine the efficacy of therapeutic interventions, including the use of assistive technology and environmental modifications, on minimizing the effects of age-related physical changes. Silverman et al. (1998) suggest that:

> aging of adults with mental retardation is associated with a complex and multidimensional set of phenomena, many aspects of

which are poorly understood at this time. Substantial investment in research, both basic and applied, will be necessary to characterize accurately the fundamental nature of lifespan development within this heterogeneous and atypical population. Prospective studies that follow the same individuals over many years are needed to provide critical documentation of the natural history of developmental aging, the clinical progression of dementing disorders, and the likelihood of occurrence of age-associated physical impairments, functional changes, and illnesses (p. 58). Research has provided information about the physical changes that accompany aging; further research is needed to determine the impact of these changes on the person at the activity, participation, and societal levels of disability.

REFERENCES

Baird, P. A., & Sadovnick, A. D. (1988). Life expectancy in Down syndrome adults. *Lancet, 330*, 1354-1356.

Braddock, D. (1999). Aging and developmental disabilities: Demographic and policy issues affecting American families. *Mental Retardation, 37*(5), 155-161.

Brzezniak, J. (1998). The effects of aging on the ambulation abilities of a developmentally disabled population. *Topics in Geriatric Rehabilitation, 13*(4), 22-29.

Burdett, C. (1998). A comparison of the health status of developmentally disabled and nondevelopmentally disabled elders. *Topics in Geriatric Rehabilitation, 13*(4), 1-11.

Burt, D., Loveland, K., Yuan-Cho, C., Chuang, A., Lewis, K., & Cherry, L. (1995). Aging in adults with Down Syndrome: Report from a longitudinal study. *American Journal on Mental Retardation, 100*(3), 262-270.

Center, J., Beange, H., & McElduff, A. (1998). People with mental retardation have an increased prevalence of osteoporosis: A population study. *American Journal on Mental Retardation, 103*(1), 19-28.

Christenson, M. A. (1990). *Aging in the designed environment.* Binghamton, NY: The Haworth Press, Inc.

Clark, F., Azen, S. P., Zemke, R., Jackson, J., Carlson, M., Mandel, D., Hay, J., Josephson, J., Cherry, B., Hessel, C., Palmer, J., & Lipson, L. (1997). Occupational therapy for independent-living older adults: A randomized controlled trial. *Journal of the American Medical Association, 278*(16), 1321-1326.

Connolly, B. H. (1998). General effects of aging on persons with developmental disabilities. *Topics in Geriatric Rehabilitation, 13*(3), 1-18.

Day, K., & Jancar, I. (1994). Mental and physical health and ageing in mental handicap: A review. *Journal of Intellectual Disability Research, 38*, 241-256.

Fenderson, C. B. (1998). Down Syndrome and aging: Implications for rehabilitation. *Topics in Geriatric Rehabilitation, 13*(4), 39-51.

Hammel, J. (2000). Assistive technology and environmental intervention (AT-EI) impact on activity and life roles of aging adults with developmental disabilities: Findings and implications for practice. *Physical & Occupational Therapy in Geriatrics, 18*(1), 37-58.

Herge, E. A., & Campbell, J. E. (1998). The role of the occupational and physical therapist in the rehabilitation of the older adult with mental retardation. *Topics in Geriatric Rehabilitation, 13*(4), 12-21.

Herr, S. S. & Weber, G. (1999). Aging and developmental disabilities. In S. S. Herr & G. Weber (Eds,). *Aging, rights, and quality of life* (pp. 1-16). Baltimore: Paul H. Brookes Publishing Co.

Hogg, J. (1997). Intellectual disability and ageing: Ecological perspectives from recent research. *Journal of Intellectual Disability Research, 41*(2), 136-143.

Hotaling, G. (1998). Rehabilitation of adults with developmental disabilities: An occupational therapy perspective. *Topics in Geriatric Rehabilitation, 13*(3), 73-83.

Janicki, M. P., Dalton, A. J., Henderson, C. M., & Davidson, P. W. (1999). Mortality and morbidity among older adults with intellectual disability: Health services considerations. *Disability and Rehabilitation, 21*(5/6), 284-294.

Jenkins, E. L., Hildreth, B. L., & Hildreth, G. (1993). Elderly persons with mental retardation: An exceptional population with special needs. *International Journal of Aging and Human Development, 37*(1), 69-80.

Lohiya, G. S., Lohiya, S., & Tan-Figuerroa, L. (1999). Eighteen fractures in a man with profound mental retardation. *Mental Retardation, 37*(1), 47-51.

Lubin, R. A., & Kiley, M. (1985). Epidemiology of aging in developmental disabilities. In M. P. Janicki & H. M. Wisniewski (Eds.), *Aging and developmental disabilities: Issues and approaches* (pp. 95-113). Baltimore: Paul H. Brookes Publishing Co.

Ludow, B. L. (1999). Life after Loss. In S. S. Herr & G. Weber (Eds,). *Aging, rights, and quality of life* (pp. 189-221). Baltimore: Paul H. Brookes Publishing Co.

Machemer, R. H., & Overeynder, J. C. (Eds.). (1993). Aging and developmental disabilities: An in-service curriculum. Rochester, NY: University of Rochester.

Mann, W. C. & Hurren, D. (1994). RERC-Aging workshop manual: Age-related changes. Buffalo, NY: State University of NY at Buffalo.

Miller, C. A. (1992). Biophysical development during late adulthood. In C. S. Schuster & S. S. Ashburn (Eds.), *The process of human development: A holistic life-span approach* (3rd ed., pp. 804-830). Philadelphia: J. P. Lippincott Company.

Moss, S. (1999). Mental health: Issues of access and quality of life. In S. S. Herr & G. Weber (Eds,). *Aging, rights, and quality of life* (pp. 167-187). Baltimore: Paul H. Brookes Publishing Co.

Murphy, K. P., Molnar, G. E., & Lankasky, K. (1995). Medical and functional status of adults with cerebral palsy. *Developmental Medicine and Child Neurology, 37*, 1075-1084.

Overeynder, J. C., & Turk, M. A. (1998). Cerebral palsy and aging: A framework for promoting the health of older persons with cerebral palsy. *Topics in Geriatric Rehabilitation, 13*(3), 19-24.

Silverman, W., Zigman, W. B., Kim, H., Krinsky-McHale, S., & Wisniewski, H. M.

(1998). Aging and dementia among adults with mental retardation and Down Syndrome. *Topics in Geriatric Rehabilitation, 13*(3), 49-64.

Strauss, D., & Eyman, R. K. (1996). Mortality of people with mental retardation in California with and without Down Syndrome, 1986-1991. *American Journal on Mental Retardation, 100,* 643-653.

U.S. Senate Special Committee on Aging (1991). *Aging America: Trends and projections 133.* Washington, D.C.: U.S. Government Printing Office.

Wagemans, A. M., Fiolet, J. F., van der Linden, E. S., & Menheere, P. P. (1998). Osteoporosis and intellectual disability: Is there any relation? *Journal of Intellectual Disability Research, 42*(5), 370-374.

WHO. (2000). *ICIDH-2: International Classification of Functioning and Disability.* Website address: http://www.who.int/icidh/index.htm (1/20/00). Geneva: World Health Organization.

Zigman, W., Silverman, W., & Wisniewski, H. M. (1996). Aging and Alzheimer's disease in Down syndrome: Clinical and pathological changes. *Mental Retardation and Developmental Disabilities Research Review, 2,* 73-79.

Overview of Health Issues of Older Women with Intellectual Disabilities

Carol J. Gill, PhD
Allison A. Brown

SUMMARY. Health researchers, educators and providers have begun to address the health needs of women and girls with disabilities in the U.S. Older women with intellectual disabilities, however, remain underrepresented in the national health research agenda. As this population becomes more visible and empowered through policies that support greater community integration and longevity, they and their families, professionals and advocates need more accurate information about their health concerns and options. A critical problem is that professionals receive little training regarding the health concerns and experiences of women with intellectual disabilities who are growing older. This paper provides an overview of primary health issues related to aging for women with intellectual disabilities in the following areas: (1) general health, (2) reproductive health, (3) mental health, and (4) access to health services. The

Carol J. Gill is Assistant Professor, Department of Disability and Human Development, University of Illinois at Chicago, Chicago, IL. Allison A. Brown is a PhD Student, School of Public Health; and Field Coordinator, Rehabilitation Research and Training Center on Aging with Mental Retardation, Department of Disability and Human Development, University of Illinois at Chicago, Chicago, IL.

Address correspondence to: Carol J. Gill, PhD, Department of Disability and Human Development (MC 626), 1640 West Roosevelt Road, Chicago, IL 60608.

This publication is sponsored in part by the Rehabilitation Research and Training Center on Aging with Mental Retardation which is funded by the National Institute on Disability and Rehabilitation Research under grant #H133B980046. The opinions contained in this document are those of the grantee and do not necessarily reflect those of the U.S. Department of Education.

[Haworth co-indexing entry note]: "Overview of Health Issues of Older Women with Intellectual Disabilities." Gill, Carol J., and Allison A. Brown. Co-published simultaneously in *Physical & Occupational Therapy in Geriatrics* (The Haworth Press, Inc.) Vol. 18, No. 1, 2000, pp. 23-36; and: *Aging and Developmental Disability: Current Research, Programming, and Practice Implications* (ed: Joy Hammel, and Susan M. Nochajski) The Haworth Press, Inc., 2000, pp. 23-36. Single or multiple copies of this article are available for a fee from The Haworth Document Delivery Service [1-800-342-9678, 9:00 a.m. - 5:00 p.m. (EST). E-mail address: getinfo@haworthpressinc.com].

paper concludes with a discussion of implications for practice and research, and recommendations for future research and health service provision for women with intellectual disabilities. *[Article copies available for a fee from The Haworth Document Delivery Service: 1-800-342-9678. E-mail address: <getinfo@haworthpressinc.com> Website: <http://www.HaworthPress. com>]*

KEYWORDS. Intellectual disabilities, mental retardation, women's health, older women, aging, developmental disabilities, health care

INTRODUCTION

The past decade has been a productive and historically important phase in women's health research, policy, education and services. Across the country, diverse yet unified voices have called for a new health agenda to reflect more accurately women's complex health experiences (Dan, 1994). The National Institutes of Health (NIH) Women's Health Initiative and other efforts resulting from this activism have begun to redress the longstanding neglect of women in research and policy (Matthews, Shumaker, Bowen, Langer, Hunt, Kaplan, Klesges & Rittenbaugh, 1997).

In contrast to the status of women in the general population, however, health research on the issues of women with disabilities has lagged behind. Historically, research on the health needs of persons with disabilities failed to attend to gender and focused primarily on men recovering from war or work-related injuries (Fine & Asch, 1988). In the 1980s and 1990s, however, women with physical and sensory disabilities started communicating their health experiences in written accounts (Campling, 1981; Duffy, 1981; Matthews, 1983) and at disability conferences (e.g., The Health of Women with Physical Disabilities Conference, Bethesda, MD, 1994; Disabled Women's Symposium, Rockville, MD, 1994 and Oakland, CA, 1995; Promoting the Health and Wellness of Women with Disabilities Conference, San Antonio, TX, 1999). They began to speak out for greater self-determination in health services and for greater public recognition of their status as women. They joined forces with specialists in rehabilitation medicine to develop research and service programs responsive to their needs. Some professional women with disabilities started conducting their own research projects.

A corpus of data on disabled women's health issues is thus beginning to form but most of it focuses on working-age women with physical disabilities. The health needs of women with intellectual disabilities have received little attention (Lunsky & Reiss, 1998). Older women with intellectual disabilities, moreover, have barely progressed to the margins of health research (Administration on Developmental Disabilities, 1998, *Federal Register,* March 30, 1998), and most existing studies concern women living in residential facilities rather than in natural settings.

This is a critical knowledge gap, particularly in light of current trends affecting citizens with intellectual disabilities. Public policies increasingly urge community integration rather than institutional placement (Ridenour & Norton, 1997). Improved healthcare, protections and supports have increased longevity in this population. As women with intellectual disabilities consequently become more visible and empowered to take their place in the community, they and their families, professionals and advocates need accurate information about their health needs and options.

Yet few professional training programs address the needs of women with intellectual disabilities, let alone the growing numbers who will reach advanced age. The lack of such training becomes more problematic as women with intellectual disabilities become more socially active, resulting in their heightened need for informed reproductive and other health services (Sulpizi, 1996). If these women continue to be overlooked, misunderstood or regarded as asexual by health care professionals (Focht-New, 1996; Sulpizi, 1996; Thornton, 1996), they are not likely to receive adequate services regarding the aging process.

More information regarding this population is critically needed by health professionals who plan clinical interventions, including therapy approaches and supports for successful community living. The remainder of this article begins to respond to this need by providing an overview of the major health issues of older women with intellectual disabilities followed by a discussion of implications for therapy and research.

BACKGROUND

Sadly, the history of health services for women with intellectual disabilities has been marked by harsh treatment and violations of self-determination. Endorsed by the Supreme Court decision in *Buck v. Bell* (1927), the forced sterilization of intellectually disabled women was once commonplace and continued into the 1970s (Prevatt, 1998). Institutionalization was routine and often encouraged by health professionals. Although current standards for informed consent offer improved protections for women with intellectual disabilities, many still undergo sterilization or long term contraception, without their assent, for the purpose of easier menstrual hygiene or the prevention of pregnancy (Elkins, Gafford, Wilks, Muram, & Golden, 1986; Prevatt, 1998). In research, they express their fears of medical procedures and report that they still endure too many encounters with health professionals who handle their bodies without asking permission or offering any explanation (Martin, Roy, Wells, & Lewis, 1997).

Fortunately, women with intellectual disabilities are finding their voices and finding their way into community life. Qualitative researchers have begun to ask for their viewpoints and experiences regarding their health needs. Health professionals are designing programs that offer information and options in a milieu of respect and care. The rights and abilities of these women to make choices are increasingly acknowledged by their families, guardians and health service providers. It is, perhaps, the best time in history for these women to mature into older age and for their professionals to develop the knowledge to support this process.

GENERAL HEALTH

It is unclear to what extent older persons with intellectual disabilities experience more health problems, or a faster rate of physical decline, than do age-matched persons in the general population (Cooper, 1999; Evenhuis, 1997; Kapell, Nightingale, Rodriguez, Lee, Zigman & Schupf, 1998; Martin et al. 1997; Ridenour & Norton, 1997). Available research has generally failed to demonstrate a consistent pattern of differences between older women and men with intellectual disabilities with respect to types and rates of common health problems. Gender differences were found in mortality-associated conditions in New York state (Janicki, Dalton, Henderson, & Davidson, 1999). According to this study, women with intellectual disabilities have a higher rate of cancer and higher rate of heart disease, but lower rates of respiratory disease than men with intellectual disabilities. In contrast, Rimmer, Braddock and Fujiura (1992) found that female participants with intellectual disabilities had better lipid profiles and a lower probability of heart disease than men. A national study of men and women with intellectual disabilities aged 63 or above living in facilities, however, demonstrated no sex differences in reported rates of high blood pressure, arthritis and heart disease (Anderson, Lakin, Bruininks & Hill, 1987). Women in this study were less likely than men to have had liver problems, brain damage and gum disease.

Residential setting may influence whether women with intellectual disabilities are at increased risk for developing heart disease. Women with intellectual disabilities who live at home with a family member ' may have higher levels of cholesterol and obesity and lower cardio-vascular fitness than the general population, which places them at greater risk for heart problems (Rimmer, Braddock & Marks, 1995). In addition, individuals with Down syndrome have a higher rate of congenital heart disease and it is unclear what impact this has on later life (Adlin, 1993) and other age-related risk factors for disease.

Data from multiple sources suggest that obesity and nutritional disorders may be a particular problem for older women with intellec-tual disabilities (Ridenour & Norton, 1997; Rimmer, Braddock & Fujiura, 1993). In the previously cited national study of persons with intellectual disabilities age 63 and over (Anderson et al. 1987), women were significantly more likely than men to have problems with mal-nutrition/obesity. There is a higher prevalence of obesity among adult women with Down syndrome (Chicoine, Rubin, & McGuire, 1997) than in the general population of adult women.

REPRODUCTIVE HEALTH

In general, women with intellectual disabilities parallel women in the general population with respect to age of onset and regularity of men-struation. For example, Scola and Pueschel (1992) found that 76% of women with Down syndrome 13-27 years of age (n = 51) had regular menstrual cycles compared with 73% of a high school population. Most menstrual cycles of women with intellectual disabilities involve ovula-tion and formation of a *corpus luteum,* suggesting that gonadal endo-crine function is within normal ranges. However, little information is available on how hormone levels and gonadal function change with age for persons with Down syndrome. Both men and women show eleva-tions of follicle-stimulating hormone (FSH) and luteinizing hormone

(LH) at puberty indicative of primary gonadal dysfunction (Schupf, Kapell, Nightingale, Rodriguez, Tycko, & Mayeux, 1998).

Prolonged use of psychotropic and anti-seizure medication is common in this population and may be associated with menstrual disruption, infertility and age-related disorders linked to reduced estrogen levels. For some women with epilepsy, menopause is associated with changes in seizure activity and may be related to new-onset of seizures occurring during or after menopause (Abbasi, Krumholz, Kittner, & Langenberg, 1999). Anderson et al. (1987) reported that slightly over 3% of older women with intellectual disabilities were characterized as having had "female problems." They and their male counterparts received high levels of antipsychotic medications (about 1 in 5). Unfortunately, little formal research has systematically examined the effects of such medications on the health of aging women with intellectual disabilities.

Several studies have discovered an earlier onset of menopause for women with Down syndrome compared to women with other intellectual disabilities and women in the general population. Carr and Hollins (1995) investigated the menstrual histories of 45 women with Down syndrome and 126 women with learning disabilities aged 36 to 61 years. They found that 87% of women with Down syndrome had stopped menstruating by the age of 46 and 100% had stopped by age 51. Among women with intellectual disabilities, 69% had stopped menstruating by age 46 and 100% had stopped by age 54. Using logistic regression, Schupf, Zigman, Kapell, Lee, Kline, and Levin (1997) determined that the age-adjusted likelihood of menopause was twice as high in women with Down syndrome as in women with other intellectual disabilities. Seltzer, Schupf, and Wu (1999) found that women with Down syndrome in their study had a median age at menopause that was 4-5 years earlier than women in the general population. The investigators conclude "Early menopause in women with Down syndrome may be both a reflection of premature or accelerated aging and a risk factor for estrogen-related disorders such as heart disease, depression, osteoporosis, breast cancer and dementia that increase in frequency following menopause. It has been suggested that older individuals with Down syndrome show age-related changes in health, cognitive and functional capacities indicative of accelerated aging . . . and early menopause would be consistent with this hypothesis."

As previously mentioned, women with intellectual disabilities may undergo hysterectomy or long term contraception, such as Norplant or hormone injections, when caregivers seek solutions to menstrual management or pregnancy prevention. Such interventions are often unnecessary and can be supplanted by appropriate education in menstrual self-care and alternative approaches to contraception (Elkins et al., 1986; Prevatt, 1997). These alternatives allow women to maintain body integrity and to choose fertility if desired. Although it is a controversial topic, many women with intellectual disabilities have successfully managed wanted pregnancies and subsequent child-rearing. Furthermore, the long term effects of the more radical contraceptive methods on aging women with intellectual disabilities has not been adequately studied. Not only is it respectful to involve women in matters affecting their own bodies, but sterilization should never be relied upon as a cure-all. It offers no protection against sexually transmitted disease or the trauma of sexual abuse. Family members and professionals have a responsibility to consider the full range of present and future hazards confronting women with intellectual disabilities when deciding on the best forms of contraception.

Some studies on persons with physical and specific developmental disabilities suggest that disability status and related treatments can significantly affect the process of aging for women. For example, preliminary reports on women with intellectual disabilities and women with physical disabilities suggest that osteoporosis may occur earlier than in the nondisabled population (Ehrenkranz & May 1993; Turk, Overeynder & Janicki, 1995), leading to an increased risk of fractures. Center, Beange and McElduff (1998) found an increased prevalence of osteoporosis in a relatively young group of females and males with intellectual disabilities, and an association of low bone density and fracture in females but not males. Although the longtime use of anticonvulsives is a known risk factor for osteoporosis for both sexes, Jancar and Jancar (1998) found that women with intellectual disabilities and epilepsy were more likely to sustain fractures than their male counterparts. Hormone replacement therapy has been used in the general population as a primary prevention for heart disease and osteoporosis, but it has not been studied systematically in this group.

MENTAL HEALTH

It has frequently been reported that persons with intellectual disabilities are at increased risk for mental health problems compared to the general population (Cooper, 1999; Holland & Koot, 1998), although direct comparisons between the two groups have not been adequately studied. Because of communication limitations, emotional problems of older women with intellectual disabilities may be difficult to diagnose until a significant behavior change occurs. A variety of causes and risk factors should be explored to account for such change, including: underlying depression, anxiety and other psychiatric illness; reactions to physical illness, pain, and hormonal fluctuations (Ridenour & Norton, 1997); feelings of grief following loss of significant relationships; and effects of abuse. Since women with intellectual disabilities, like women in general, are likely to live longer than their male counterparts, they may be more likely to experience the loss of family members and other key supporters as they age.

Dementia is common in older persons with intellectual disabilities, occurring at about four times the rate found in the age-matched general population (Cooper, 1999). For example, Down syndrome has been associated with early onset Alzheimer's disease; however, postmenopausal women with Down syndrome appear to be significantly less likely to acquire Alzheimer's disease than their male counterparts (Schupf et al., 1998).

Varied sources indicate that women with intellectual disabilities experience high rates of physical and sexual abuse, a risk factor for the development of depression, anxiety and other psychiatric disorders. Typically, the perpetrators are known by the women and are frequently relatives or others who provide assistance or services, such as direct care staff or attendants (Lumley & Miltenberger, 1997). Factors thought to increase risk for this population include difficulty communicating, lack of adequate sex education, and inadequate social skills training. Although there is evidence that self-protection skills training can be effective, little research has investigated the relative effectiveness of abuse prevention and intervention strategies. Additionally, health care providers and other staff may lack sensitivity to the risk of abuse for women with intellectual disabilities. For example, Kopac, Fritz, and Holt (1998) reported that over a third of service provider agencies included in their study indicated that questions related to the identification and treatment of sexual abuse for women with developmental disabilities were not applicable to their agencies.

Depending on the cause, mental health problems of older women with intellectual disabilities can be addressed through interventions such as supportive counseling, increased opportunities for meaningful activities, and treatment of underlying pain and illness. Although psychotropic medications have been historically overused in managing behavior problems in persons with intellectual disabilities, judicious use of these agents may be helpful to some individuals.

ACCESS TO HEALTH SERVICES

The likelihood that women with intellectual disabilities will receive routine health exams, particularly reproductive health exams, is complicated by several factors. The need for such services may be overlooked by healthcare professionals, family members, and legal guardians who fail to consider the sexuality and gender-related needs of this group. As previously mentioned, few physicians and other health professionals receive adequate training regarding the health issues of women with intellectual disabilities, including ways to facilitate medical examinations. Consequently, professionals may avoid providing services to this population. Obtaining informed consent for health services can be complicated by diminished comprehension of many women with intellectual disabilities. The pressures of managed care funding may severely compromise the time needed for sensitive and respectful procedures. Transportation problems can be a barrier to getting to appointments at all. Furthermore, women with intellectual disabilities often have related physical disabilities that are not well accommodated in inaccessible medical service settings.

Data on access to health services for older women with intellectual disabilities are scant. The National Medical Expenditure Survey (1987) included a very small sample (N = 19) of women with intellectual disabilities age 40 and above. Results suggested that these women may not be receiving adequate reproductive health services. Only 20% had received a pap smear within the past year, an additional 26% had received one within two years, 58% had received one more than two years ago, and 16% had never had one. Approximately one-fourth had never received a breast examination. Only 15% had ever had a mammogram (Anderson, 1996). Edgerton, Gaston, Kelly, and Ward (1994) found that very few of the women in their 5 year ethnographic study had received a mammogram or pap smear. Included in the sample was a woman who had developed breast cancer and another woman who had developed cancer of the uterus, neither of whom had ever received a prior preventive screening related to their cancer. Consistent with findings in the United States, Stein and Allen (1999) also reported in their study of 389 British women with learning (intellectual) disabilities that cervical cancer screening for women with intellectual disabilities is significantly lower than for the general female population.

Several authors have described various approaches, strategies and models for the provision of health services, particularly reproductive health services, to women with intellectual disabilities (Elkins et al., 1986; Prevatt, 1998; Whitmore, 1999). Unfortunately, many women in this group are still not receiving basic routine healthcare because of insurance gaps, health professionals' lack of knowledge about and willingness to treat this population, perceived difficulty in obtaining informed consent, and the women's fears of examinations and other medical procedures. Available services vary in their responsiveness to the women's needs. For example, programs that use cooperative strategies with the women emphasizing straightforward information, education, and progressive desensitization regarding medical procedures have reported success in service delivery with this population. Yet it is common to see sedation and even general anaesthesia used routinely to conduct reproductive health exams in women who fear them. Although such approaches may be necessary as a last resort for some individuals, they should not be employed simply to save time or to circumvent a thorough effort to gain informed consent. Used to excess, these strategies merely reinforce the women's fears and loss of control in the medical setting.

IMPLICATIONS FOR PRACTICE AND RESEARCH

Physically, psychologically and socially, the current status of older women with intellectual disabilities is interesting but not yet well described empirically. As these women live longer and leave institutional life behind, health professionals will increasingly meet them in their practices. The data reviewed above suggest the following:

1. Possible earlier onset and heightened risk for health problems in this population must be considered when designing exercise programs, activities and other interventions. Although increased activity can help counteract the harmful effects of unhealthy diet and sedentary lifestyle, such changes must be implemented with caution.

2. Whenever possible, it is beneficial to involve the individual in the design and direction of her program. The abilities and needs for self-determination in older women with intellectual disabilities have been routinely underestimated as resources to be utilized in therapy.

3. Attention to communication and education is critical. Many older women with disabilities can express their needs, concerns and preferences when given an opportunity. In turn, they want to be informed about their options and about what they can expect to happen to them.

4. The role(s) of family and agency care providers should not be underestimated. Individuals who provide primary support to older women with disabilities can be effective in facilitating opportunities for women with disabilities to have safe and appropriate health experiences, and in supporting them to develop their own personal health promotion practices.

5. It is important to focus on the fact that older women with intellectual disabilities are women. They have a full array of reproductive health needs. Most of them need information about aging, their bodies and sexuality. They may wish access to roles and options, such as someone's girlfriend or having uninterrupted periods, that others might summarily dismiss as inappropriate for this group.

6. Abuse and mental health problems must be acknowledged as issues that are equal to physical problems in importance. If women cannot readily communicate their needs in this area, their health professionals must remain attentive to clues that signal a need for support or intervention.

7. In terms of research, the issues of this population present an open vista. More research is needed on the rates and prevalence of physical and mental health conditions, including comparisons with the general population and with both men and younger women with intellectual disabilities. Preventive healthcare programs need to be developed and tested for effectiveness. Educational programs on health, sexuality and abuse must be designed for the women themselves and for their families and professionals. Innovative research designs should incorporate participatory strategies that allow older women with disabilities to contribute their critical perspectives to this knowledge base.

REFERENCES

Abbasi, F., Krumholz, A., Kittner, S. J. & Langenberg, P. (1999). Effects of menopause on seizures in women with epilepsy. *Epilepsia, 40*, (2):205-210.

Anderson, D. J. (1996). Health-related needs and services for older adults with MR/DD. Symposium presented at *American Association on Mental Retardation*, San Antonio, Texas, June, 1996.

Anderson, D., Lakin, K., Bruininks, R. & Hill, B. (1987). *A National Study of Residential and Support Services for Elderly Persons with Mental Retardation.* Minneapolis, MN: University of Minnesota.

Campling, J. (1981). (Ed.). *Images of ourselves: Disabled women talking.* Boston: Routledge & Kegan Paul.

Carr, J. & Hollins, S. (1995). Menopause in women with learning disabilities. *Journal of Intellectual Disability Research, 39*, (Pt 2):137-139.

Chicoine, B., Rubin, S., & McGuire, D. (1997). *Health and psychosocial findings of the Adult Mental Retardation Center.* Presentation at the International Roundtable on Aging and Intellectual Disability, Chicago, IL.

Cooper, S. A. (1999). The relationship between psychiatric and physical health in elderly people with intellectual disability. *Journal of Intellectual Disability Research, 43*, 54-60.

Dan, A. J. (1994). (Ed.) *Reframing Women's Health.* Thousand Oaks, CA: Sage Publications.

Duffy, Y. (1981). . . . *All things are possible.* Ann Arbor, MI: A. J. Garvin Assoc.

Edgerton, R. B., Gaston, M. A., Kelly, H., & Ward, T. W. (1994). Health care for aging people with mental retardation. *Mental Retardation, 32*, (2): 146-150.

Elkins, T. E., Gafford, L. S., Wilks, C. S. Muram, D. & Golden, G. (1986). A model clinic approach to the reproductive health concerns of the mentally handicapped. *Obstetrics & Gynecology, 68*, (2), 185-188.

Evenhuis, H. M. (1997). Medical aspects of ageing in a population with intellectual disability: III. Mobility, internal conditions and cancer. *Journal of Intellectual Disability Research, 41*, (Pt 1): 8-18.

Fine, M. & Asch, A. (1988). (Eds). *Women with disabilities: Essays in psychology, culture, and politics.* Philadelphia, PA, USA: Temple University Press.

Focht-New, V. (1996). Beyond abuse: health care for people with disabilities. *Issues in Mental Health Nursing, 17*, (5): 427-438.

Goodenough, G. K. & Hole-Goodenough, J. (1997). Training for primary care of mentally handicapped patients in US family practice residencies. *Journal of the American Board of Family Practice, 10*, (5): 333-336.

Holland, A. J. & Koot, H. M. (1998). Mental health and intellectual disability: An international perspective. *Journal of Intellectual Disability Research, 42*, 505-512.

Jancar, J. & Jancar, M. P. (1998). Age-related fractures in people with intellectual disability and epilepsy. *Journal of Intellectual Disability Research, 42* (Pt 5): 429-433.

Janicki, M. P., Dalton, A. J., Henderson, C. M. & Davidson, P. W. (1999). Mortality and morbidity among older adults with intellectual disability: Health services considerations. *Disability and Rehabilitation, 21*,(5-6): 284-294.

Kapell, D., Nightingale, B., Rodriguez, A., Lee J. H., Zigman, W. B. & Schupf, N. (1998). Prevalence of chronic medical conditions in adults with mental retardation: Comparison with the general population. *Mental Retardation, 36,* (4): 269-279.

Kopac, C. A., Fritz J. & Holt R. A. (1998). Gynecologic and reproductive services for women with developmental disabilities. *Clinical Excellence for Nurse Practitioners, 2,* (2):88-95.

Lumley, V. A. & Miltenberger, R. G. (1997). Sexual abuse prevention for persons with mental retardation. *American Journal on Mental Retardation, 101,* (5), 459-472.

Lunsky, Y. & Reiss, S. (1998). Health needs of women with mental retardation and developmental disabilities. *American Psychologist, 53,* 319.

Martin, D. M., Roy, A., Wells, R. B., & Lewis, J. (1997). Health gain through screening-users' and carers' perspectives of health care: Developing primary health care services for people with an intellectual disability. *Journal of Intellectual & Developmental Disability, 22,* (4), 241-242.

Matfhews, G. F. (1983). *Voices from the shadows: Women with disabilities speak out.* Toronto: Women's Educational Press.

Matthews, K. A., Shumaker, S. A., Bowen, D. J., Langer, R. D., Hunt, J. R., Kaplan, R. M., Klesges, R. M., & Rittenbaugh, C. (1997). Women's health initiative: Why now? What is it? What's new? *American Psychologist, 52,* 101-116.

Prevatt, B. (1998). Gynecologic care for women with mental retardation. *Journal of Obstetric, Gynecologic, & Neonatal Nursing, 7,* (3), 2516.

Ridenour, N. & Norton, D. (1997). Community-based persons with mental retardation: Opportunities for health promotion. *Nurse Practitioner Forum, 8,* (2), 45-49.

Rimmer, J. H., Braddock, D. & Fujiura, G. (1992). Blood lipid and percent body fat levels in Down syndrome versus non-DS persons with mental retardation. *Adapted Physical Activity Quarterly, 9,* (2): 123-129.

Rimmer, J. H., Braddock, D. & Fujiura, G. (1993). Prevalence of obesity in adults with mental retardation: Implications for health promotion and disease prevention. *Mental Retardation, 31,* (2): 105-110.

Rimmer, J. H., Braddock, D. & Marks, B. (1995). Health characteristics and behaviors of adults with mental retardation residing in three living arrangements. *Research in Developmental Disabilities, 16,* (6): 489-499.

Seltzer, G. B., Schupf, N. & Wu, H. (1999). A prospective study of menopause in women with Down syndrome. Manuscript submitted for publication.

Schupf, N., Kapell, D., Nightingale, B., Rodriguez, A., Tycko, B. & Mayeux, R. (1998). Earlier onset of Alzheimer's disease in men with Down syndrome. *Neurology, 50* (4): 991-995.

Schupf, N., Zigman, W., Kapell, D., Lee, J. H., Kline, J. & Levin, B. (1997). Early menopause in women with Down's syndrome. *Journal of Intellectual Disability Research, 41,* (Pt 3): 264-267.

Scola, P. S. & Pueschel, S. M. (1992). Menstrual cycles and basal body temperature curves in women with Down syndrome. *Obstetrics and Gynecology, 79,* (1): 91-94.

Stein, K. & Allen, N. (1999). Cross sectional survey of cervical cancer screening in women with learning disability. *British Medical Journal, 318*, (7184): 641.

Sulpizi, L. K. (1996). Issues in sexuality and gynecologic care of women with developmental disabilities. *Journal of Obstetric, Gynecologic, & Neonatal Nursing, 25*, (7):609-614.

Thornton, C. (1996). A focus group inquiry into the perceptions of primary health care teams and the provision of health care for adults with a learning disability living in the community. *Journal of Advanced Nursing, 23*, (6): 1168-1176.

Turk, M. A., Overeynder, J. C. & Janicki, M. P. (1995). Uncertain Future-Aging and Cerebral Palsy: Clinical Concerns. Albany. NY: New York State Developmental Disabilities Planning Council.

Whitmore, J. (1999). Cervical screening for women with learning disability. Sefton has multidisciplinary group to promote sexual health care for these women. *British Medical Journal, 318*, (7182): 537.

Assistive Technology and Environmental Intervention (AT-EI) Impact on the Activity and Life Roles of Aging Adults with Developmental Disabilities: Findings and Implications for Practice

Joy Hammel, PhD, OTR/L, FAOTA

SUMMARY. As persons age with developmental disabilities, they experience life long disability and age-related issues at the impairment, activity, participation and environment levels. Assistive technology and environmental interventions (AT-EI) can serve as potential mediators in delaying or preventing functional decline, health conditions, and dependent care placements only if they are considered within the dynamic interaction of the person, activities, and the facilitators and barriers within the social and physical environment. This paper summarizes AT-EI needs, research results, and implications for practice specific to persons with developmental disabilities, and important others in their lives, as they age in place. *[Article copies available for a fee from The Haworth Document Delivery Service: 1-800-342-9678. E-mail address: <getinfo@haworth pressinc.com> Website: <http://www.HaworthPress.com>]*

Joy Hammel is Assistant Professor, Occupational Therapy Department, University of Illinois at Chicago, 1919 West Taylor Street, Room 311, Chicago, IL 60612 (E-mail: hammel@uic.edu).

Preparation of this article was supported in part by funding from the Rehabilitation Research and Training Center on Aging with Mental Retardation, University of Illinois at Chicago, through the U.S. Department of Education, National Institute on Disability and Rehabilitation Research, Grant number H133B980046. The opinions contained in this publication are those of the grantee and do not necessarily reflect those of the U.S. Department of Education.

[Haworth co-indexing entry note]: "Assistive Technology and Environmental Intervention (AT-EI) Impact on the Activity and Life Roles of Aging Adults with Developmental Disabilities: Findings and Implications for Practice." Hammel, Joy. Co-published simultaneously in *Physical & Occupational Therapy in Geriatrics* (The Haworth Press, Inc.) Vol. 18, No. 1, 2000, pp. 37-58; and: *Aging and Developmental Disability: Current Research, Programming, and Practice Implications* (ed: Joy Hammel, and Susan M. Nochajski) The Haworth Press, Inc., 2000, pp. 37-58. Single or multiple copies of this article are available for a fee from The Haworth Document Delivery Service [1-800-342-9678, 9:00 a.m. - 5:00 p.m. (EST). E-mail address: getinfo@haworthpressinc.com].

KEYWORDS. Assistive technology, environmental intervention, developmental disability, mental retardation, intellectual disabilities, aging, research

INTRODUCTION

Assistive technology and environmental interventions (AT-EI) can impact upon impairment, function, living situation, and quality of life of people with disabilities across the lifespan. As persons age in place, AT-EI has been shown to delay functional decline and costs related to institutionalization (Mann, Ottenbacher, Fraas, Tomita & Granger, 1999); however much less is known about the impact of these interventions upon persons with lifelong disabilities who are aging in place. This is especially true for persons with developmental disabilities, such as mental retardation, autism, and cerebral palsy, who may experience the combined effects of disability, long term medication use, and aging, in conjunction with changes in their physical environments and social support systems. Societal barriers related to funding of resources to support community living (e.g., technology, home modifications), and stereotypes about the perceived need for and benefit of AT-EI as one ages further complicate service delivery.

A person's interaction with his physical and social environment greatly impacts upon whether or not AT-EI are accepted and integrated within everyday life, or instead, rejected, minimally utilized, or not even considered. This article examines this interaction between aging adults with developmental disabilities, their social supports, and AT-EI that could serve as community living tools for both.

The Need: There are an estimated 526,000 people over age 60 with mental retardation and other developmental disabilities in the United States; this number is predicted to double by the year 2030 (Heller & Factor, 1998). As summarized by Nochajski (2000), normative aging may involve motor, perceptual, sensory and cognitive changes that may or may not impact upon functional performance. Research suggests that people with developmental disabilities may experience these changes earlier than the nondisabled population (Jacobson & Janicki, 1983; Janicki & MacEachron, 1984; Janicki, Otis, Puccio, Rettig & Jacobson, 1985).

The majority of persons with developmental disabilities live in the community; 51% live with family members or in homes with 1-6 people. The remainder live in community group homes or supported living situations with 7-15 people (14%) (Braddock, Hemp, Parish & Westrich, 1998). Despite this level of community integration, 10% continue to live in nursing homes, and 26% live in settings of 16 or more people, such as Intermediate Care Facilities (ICFs) or institutions, thus representing diverse settings with diverse expectations for function and participation.

Over 13 million people with disabilities, with increasing rates among older adults, use AT or modify their home environments to accommodate age and disability-related issues while aging (LaPlante, Hendershot & Moss, 1992; Russell, Hendershot, LeClere, & Howie, 1997). According to the definitions used within the Developmental Disabilities Assistance and Bill of Rights Act (1994; currently undergoing reauthorization), AT is "any item, piece of equipment, or product system, whether acquired commercially, modified or customized, that is used to increase, maintain, or improve functional capabilities of individuals with developmental disabilities." The Act goes on to define AT services as: assessing function in the individual's customary environment; selecting, designing, fitting, customizing, adapting, applying, maintaining, repairing or replacing AT; coordinating and using other therapies, interventions, or services with AT; and training or technical assistance with the consumer, caregivers, and important others involved in their life. Given these definitions, it is clear that AT-EI can be used by therapists as functional tools within later life planning, programming and living situation decisions with aging persons with developmental disabilities and their caregivers.

In some states, AT-EI has been legally mandated through class action suits on behalf of persons with developmental disabilities to support transitions to the community, or to maintain health and quality of life within dependent care settings (Presperin Pedersen, 1995). However, AT-EI often is not considered or provided to this population unless therapists justify the need and tie such interventions to health, functional performance, and life course planning outcomes.

In summary, there is a significant population of people with developmental disabilities who are aging in place at the same time as their caregivers. The implications for service delivery are many; this article will focus upon those related to AT-EI. Specifically, the paper focuses on AT-EI with persons with intellectual, or a combination of intellectual, sensory, communication and physical impairments that are manifest before age 22, are likely to continue indefinitely, and result in substantial functional limitations in three or more life activities and roles, including self care, language, learning, mobility, self direction, independent living, and economic self sufficiency (Developmental Disabilities Act, 1994).

There is a critical role for occupational and physical therapists to *collaborate with* people with developmental disabilities and their important others (e.g., family, caregivers, social supports, case managers, staff, and others) to:

- identify changing needs and goals of both the consumer and the caregivers as they age,
- screen for early signs of aging, additional impairment, or functional decline with referral to specialists (e.g., vision, hearing, medical, rehabilitative) as indicated,
- consult on the design and implementation of individual and community-based programs to address or delay functional decline, including AT provision and training, environmental assessment and adaptation, accessible health and wellness programming (e.g., exercise, community mobility, social activities), and information resources to support aging in place (e.g., Department on Aging, Centers for Independent Living, self advocacy groups, Internet sites, technology user groups and product vendors),
- consult with specialists to ensure that offices, equipment and services are accessible,
- consult with policy and funding agencies (e.g., housing, transportation, in-home support, technology, health care) and others (engineers, architects and designers) to allocate resources to create environments, technologies, and programs that are accessible, inclusive, meaningful, age appropriate, and encourage activity and accommodate people's functional and social needs as they age in place.

To assume these roles and justify funding and provision of these services, therapists need to understand the effects of aging and disability-related processes, and the impact of the physical environment, assistive technologies, and social support systems on the functional performance and life role choices of aging adults with developmental disabilities.

METHOD

To organize findings and practice implications, the author utilized the International Classification of Functioning and Disability (ICIDH-2) (WHO, 2000). ICIDH-2 is an international classification schema designed to provide a common language for assessing and researching functional states associated with health status. The schema focuses on the relationship between four areas: body structure and function (or impairments), activities (or activity limitations), participation (or participation restrictions), and environmental factors (or barriers) as they impact upon functioning. Table 1 summarizes current definitions, assessment strategies, and examples of issues within each that may be targeted or impacted upon within AT-EI interventions for aging adults with developmental disabilities (readers are referred to the ICIDH-2 website (*http://www.who.int/icidh/index.htm*) to examine the current schema under development, component details, and additional examples).

Following is a summary of findings related to AT-EI practice considerations across the ICIDH-2 levels with implications for service delivery and research.

FINDINGS AND PRACTICE IMPLICATIONS

Body Structure and Function Findings and Practice Implications

Body structure and function focuses upon body organs and components, and their physiological and psychological functions. Problems in body function or structure are referred to as impairments (WHO, 2000). We are quickly gaining knowledge of body structure and function changes affiliated with normative and disability-related changes as one ages, many of which have implications for AT-EI. We know less about the interaction of lifelong impairments related to developmental disability, effects of long term medication use, and normative aging processes (Nochajski, 2000; Gill & Brown, 2000). Following are brief summaries of these impairment level trends that have most relevance to AT-EI (the reader is referred to Nochajski, 2000, and Connolly, 1998, for more detailed summaries). Since this population is fairly heterogeneous in type and extent of impairments, living situation, and level of social support available, any AT-EI interventions at this level must be linked to the functional activity and participation levels if they are to be fully implemented and integrated long term.

TABLE 1. ICIDH-2 Classification Schema of Functioning and Disability as Applied to AT-EI Service Delivery and Outcomes with Aging Adults with Developmental Disabilities

	Definition	AT/EI Examples	Methods to Assess or Research Impact
Body structures and functions	**Body structures** are anatomical parts of the body such as organs, limbs and their components. **Body functions** are the physiological or psychological functions of body systems. **Impairments** are problems in body function or structure as a significant deviation or loss.	• Seating/positioning system to address pressure sores, spinal curvature or tone • AT to address loss or impaired movement (e.g., cane, walkers, wheelchairs) • Glasses, hearing aids, vision/hearing devices and environmental modifications • Orientation calendars, wandering monitors, safety monitors, sensory/cognitive home modifications	• Medical tests of respiratory, cardiovascular, skin integrity, neuromuscular, orthopedic, digestive, and genitourinary systems and functions • Motor tests: range, strength/force, accuracy/reliability, spasticity, endurance • Sensory testing: taste, smell, touch, pressure, position sense, etc. • Vision and hearing/vestibular testing • Perceptual testing • Cognitive assessments (e.g., orientation, attention, arousal, memory, executive functions) • Speech and language assessments • Mental/psychiatric and behavioral assessments
Activity	**Activity** is the performance of a task or action by an individual. **Activity limitations** are difficulties in performance of activities.	• AAC system for functional communication • Daily living equipment and home modifications to increase ADL/IADL independence • Adapted computer for school or work activites • Seating and mobility to improve eating, transferring and public transportation use	• Basic and Instrumental ADL/Community Living: Functional Independence Measure (FIM)(UDSMR, 1993), Assessment of Motor and Process Skills (AMPS) (Fisher, 1997); Inventory for Client and Agency Planning (ICAP) (Bruinks et al., 1986); Craig Handicap Assessment Reporting Technique (CHART) (Whiteneck et al., 1992); Kohlman Evaluation of Living Skills (Kohlman, 1992) • Educational activity assessments • Essential job duty assessments
Environment	**Environmental Factors** make up the physical, social and attitudinal environment in which people live and conduct their lives.	• ADA audits and home, worksite and community accessibility interventions • Universal design of products and living spaces • Create/refer to funding and system information resource and advocacy/legal assistance programs	• Technology need/match assessments (e.g., Scherer, 1991) • QA and consumer satisfaction surveys • Physical accessibility and safety assessments (home, work, community) (e.g., SAFER Tool) (Oliver et al., 1993) • Family, social support and physical assistance • Systems analyses (e.g., funding, housing, transportation, etc.) • Societal, cultural, and attitudinal assessments
Participation	**Participation** is an individual's involvement in life situations in relation to Health Conditions, Body Functions or Structures, Activities, and Contextual Factors. **Participation Restrictions** are problems an individual may have in the manner or extent of involvement in life situations.	• Integrated AT-EM to move to community • Consumer, family, and caregiver AT/EM trainings and long term support • Community, group and nursing home inservices on AT need and use • Cost benefit analysis of workplace reasonable accommodation	• Occupational assessments: Canadian Occupational Performance Measure (Law et al., 1994), Occupational Performance History Interview (Kielhofner et al., 1998) • Participation assessments (e.g., CHART) • Quality of Life assessments • Role assessments • Cost benefit and cost effectiveness analyses (cost to benefit ratio)

[1]Categories and definitions are from the International Classification of Functioning and Disability (ICIDH-2), current draft at http://www.who.int/icidh/ (WHO, 2000).

Sensory Issues

1. Vision: Age-related changes in vision can affect visual field integrity, dark/light change adaptation and sensitivity to light or glare, color detection, and ocular motor changes in convergence and gaze (Miller, 1992). Conditions such as glaucoma, macular degeneration, diabetic retinopathy and cataracts also increasingly occur as one ages, further impacting upon vision field, central and peripheral vision, and acuity (Miller, 1992). For aging adults with developmental disabilities, vision changes and impairments may go uncorrected or unidentified more often due to an inability to communicate them effectively to family, and limited access to specialists (Connolly, 1998). If overlooked, vision problems may be interpreted as mobility, cognitive, learning or behavioral problems.

There are a range of AT-EI to accommodate impaired or lost vision, including magnifiers, text and screen enlargers, room and task lighting, color and contrast adjustments, tactile cues and environmental markers, and products that speak or give auditory feedback. The University of New York at Buffalo's Center on Aging and Technology (website: *http://wings.buffalo.edu/ot/cat/age-older.htm*) disseminates resource and educational materials describing many visual AT-EI. Despite availability, surveys of persons with mental retardation show that few AT-EI are considered or used other than eye glasses (Wehmeyer, 1995; 1998), suggesting that service providers are not screening for these issues, or do not have information on how to address them.

2. Hearing: Between 25-40% of people over 65 have some hearing loss (Bess, Lichtenstein, & Logan, 1991). Common causes of hearing loss for aging adults with developmental disabilities include presbycusis, acute or chronic ear diseases such as otitis media, and excess wax build-up (Connolly, 1998). If left undetected or untreated, they also may manifest as mobility, balance or motor control problems; cognitive attention or response delays; and decreased socialization or emotional reactions given difficulty receiving and responding to incoming information. These issues affect level of participation in AT-EI assessments, ability to understand AT-EI training, and ability to use any AT-EI products with auditory features.

As with vision, there are many products to accommodate hearing loss, including amplifiers, vibrating devices, devices to reduce background noise, microphones to focus incoming sounds, and visual cues and signage. Hearing aids are the most frequently used hearing AT-EI among adults with developmental disabilities; however, they often are not tolerated or used routinely given aesthetics, setup, and maintenance issues (Connolly, 1998).

If hearing and/or vision loss are not screened and adequately addressed as people age, service providers may incorrectly issue mobility, cognitive, or communication AT-EI that may not address these underlying sensory issues. They also may recommend premature dependent care placements given the client's inability to process and respond to incoming information.

Therapists may be the first service providers to identify hearing and vision changes or loss during therapy sessions or AT-EI assessment. Therapists can collaborate with the client and family to provide behavioral and functional data to medical, vision and hearing specialists who may not be as familiar with the client's changing needs. They also may be involved in helping specialists ensure access to vision and hearing assessment equipment. For example, a portable phoropter that can be easily rolled around a wheelchair was designed to allow ophthalmologists to perform accessible eye exams in the community (Bidwell, 1999).

Without training and support in developing a routine to use sensory AT-EI, especially glasses and hearing aides, products are often lost or not routinely used, potentially leading to more serious outcomes such as social isolation. Therapists can help create equipment set-up, training and routine maintenance instructions to increase everyday use.

3. Somatosensory Function: Somatosensory aging changes can include decreased touch, pressure, and position sense (Connolly, 1998), all of which are critical to functional AT-EI use. For example, touch and pressure impact upon accurate and safe operation of computer, communication, and mobility technology. If the person cannot feel if they have activated a button or switch, another means of communicating that information to them, such as auditory or visual cues, is needed or they may inadvertently activate a device without knowing it.

Lower extremity position sense loss can result in increased safety and fall risk, thus implicating the need for environmental adaptations; seating, positioning and/or mobility technology; and strategy development. However, major changes in positioning and mobility, such as moving from ambulating to a wheelchair, or changing a person's position in space through a new positioning system, can significantly disrupt the person's overall static and dynamic perception of their body and the world around them. As a result, they may experience dizziness, nausea, decreased tolerance, and behavioral reactions, especially if they are unable to communicate these issues to others. Such problems can result in premature immobility or dependent mobility if not considered during such significant AT-EI changes.

4. Motor Changes: There are many issues affecting movement as one ages. Loss of flexibility can result from osteoporosis, arthritis, deconditioning, and poor nutrition (Connolly, 1998). Muscle mass, strength, coordination and speed of contraction decreases with decreased physical activity (Rice, 1989). Upper back kyphosis, flattening of the lumbar lordosis, and increased flexion at the hips and knees increasingly occur with aging, and can interact with life long scoliosis, tonal issues, and seizure disorders for aging adults with developmental disabilities (Trieschmann, 1987). Gait and balance also are affected by decreased sensory input, vestibular processing, motor control and motor output.

Orthopedic issues, such as osteoarthritis and osteoporosis, have been found to occur earlier in people with neuromotor problems who are nonambulatory or more sedentary (Mazess, 1987; Walz, Harper & Wilson, 1986). Cardiac and pulmonary function declines further limit mobility and activity. These age and disability-related motoric issues can begin a cyclical process involving increased pain, decreased endurance, further activity limitation, and increased susceptibility to injuries, such as fractures or contractures (Trieschmann, 1987).

For persons with mild to moderate mental retardation, motoric problems may be experienced as early as 50 (Janicki & Jacobsen, 1986). They may manifest as slow declines over time, or rather abrupt loss of mobility, with implications for transitioning from independent ambulation, to assisted ambulation with a walker, to independent or dependent mobility systems. Mobility and fall risk are primary factors for determining living situation. Later life screenings by therapists can detect these mobility changes and also support the consumer's ability to maintain her living situation.

In many cases, positioning and mobility problems may be due to a complex set of factors that may be beyond the scope of the primary OT or PT. In these cases, therapists can assist by getting a doctor's referral to a seating and mobility specialist, many of whom are therapists with extensive expertise in this area. These specialists may work with specialized rehabilitation technology suppliers (RTS) to assess needs, prepare specialized funding justifications, create custom solutions, and provide installation and training. Organizations such as RESNA (*http://www.resna.org/*) can link therapists to community specialists and information resources and continuing education opportunities to increase knowledge and skills.

5. *Cognitive Issues:* Whether older adults experience declines in cognitive function, and to what extent or in what areas, remains controversial and represents a large area of ongoing research. Prior studies have shown decreasing ability of older adults to adapt to new information and develop new encoding strategies to handle complex information, especially given decreased speed and accuracy in perception and psychomotor responses. However, studies also have shown that learning and cognition is greatly influenced by the structure, difficulty, meaning and interest in the activity at hand, and the environment in which it is conducted (Carr & Shepherd, 1992; Mathiowetz & Haugen, 1994; Poon et al., 1986). These findings have implications for AT-EI service provision, particularly for persons with long term intellectual impairments.

First and foremost, AT-EI assessment, intervention and training need to be done within everyday contexts with a focus on activities that are age appropriate and meaningful to the person, and his needs, interests, and social reference group. This is especially true for older adults with intellectual disabilities who have practiced behavioral strategies, routines and habits embedded in familiar environments over a lifetime.

Assessments that attempt to evaluate cognition or perceptual motor processing out of context for AT-EI decisions lack ecological validity (Poon et al., 1986). They are especially problematic for individuals with multiple impairments that interfere with valid cognitive testing. Grounding AT-EI assessment in activities gives a more valid and holistic picture of the person's abilities and capacity to integrate AT-EI into everyday life.

Secondly, unless the consumer and family have had previous exposure to AT, it can be perceived as strange, unfamiliar, ugly and even frightening. At minimum, it is certainly novel. Often, people do not have anything in their experience with which to compare it, except societal stereotypes about AT as a negative symbol of dependence. Older adults and their caregivers may choose not to use the AT-EI (Gitlin, Levine & Geiger, 1993; Gitlin, Schemm, Landsberg & Burgh, 1996), in part because it is perceived as a sign of helplessness or loss of control, or as something that does not fit into their social world. Repeated demonstrations of how to use AT-EI features to perform everyday activities within familiar settings can help increase the meaning, and decrease the frustration or fear for users. Opportunities to rent or borrow the technology to try out in the home and community are especially important. Matching the AT-EI to the existing values, interests, and routines in the home and contexts in which they will use it also is critical.

Thirdly, AT can become very complex very quickly. It is not at all uncommon to exceed cognitive limits when instructing a client and caregivers in how to use a single piece of technology, such as a power wheelchair. Making significant changes in the environment also can significantly disrupt meaning and personal routines. Coupled with this, training in use of AT-EI is often provided on a limited basis. Therapists can address these issues by:

- Selecting AT-EI with the most intuitive, user-friendly interface that can be adjusted for complexity by enabling/disabling features over time.
- Arranging more frequent yet shorter training sessions, with follow-up practice opportunities after the therapist has left, to build AT-EI problem solving skills over time.
- Stepping through set-up and troubleshooting strategies with the client and important others, with return demonstration to ensure competence.
- Providing "cheat sheets" and check lists (in verbal, print and/or picture/photographic formats) on AT-EI set-up and maintenance procedures, steps for common procedures (e.g., changing a setting such as speed) and troubleshooting (e.g., battery is dead, computer doesn't start, someone changed the environment) that can be used across multiple caregivers across the day. These instructions can be created on the computer (using word processing, databases of picture sets or clip art, digitized photos), printed, laminated, and carried in a small notebook across settings.
- Connecting AT-EI users and caregivers to information and support resources, such as other local users, vendors, information and advocacy programs (e.g., Technical Assistance Projects, Alliance for Technology Access), product and information web sites (e.g., Closing the Gap), and ways to stay current, post questions and share coping strategies.

Activity Findings and Practice Implications

The ICIDH-2 activity level (WHO, 2000) is one of the richest areas for demonstrating the need and justifying the outcomes of AT-EI for aging adults with developmental disabilities. AT-EI can impact upon *independence, safety and efficiency* in performing basic (e.g., eating, bathing, toileting) and instrumental (e.g., meal preparation, community mobility, shopping) activities of daily living. Such evidence is especially useful since AT-EI services and funding are often tied to functional impact.

Mann et al.'s (1999) randomized controlled trial of 104 frail older adults provides a powerful example of the functional impact of AT-EI upon older adults. In this study, half of the subjects received intensive, functionally-based, AT-EI services; half served as a control and received "usual" care. Although both groups experienced functional declines by 18 months post, subjects in the treatment group showed significantly less decline, and reported lower levels of pain. Although subjects in the treatment group spent more money on AT-EI products and services, those in the control group had significantly more costly expenditures for in-home nursing and case manager visits, and subsequent institutional care. Such a study strongly supports a maintenance and preventative role for functionally-based AT-EI with older adults.

Despite the benefits, recent survey results show that only a small percentage of adults with mental retardation use AT-EI, and they and their caregivers express many unmet AT-EI needs related to functional communication (10% using; 12.5% need), mobility (9% using; 7.5% need), and independent living/environmental control (7% using; 16.25% need) (Wehmeyer 1995, 1998). Of those who could potentially use common household appliances, a large percentage were not using a can opener (44%), toaster (38%), VCR (34%), radio/stereo (28%), or television (18%), even though these devices can be adapted for access with technology, environmental modifications or adaptive strategy training.

Two descriptive studies have examined the functional impact of AT-EI interventions with aging adults with developmental disabilities. In the first study, 35 persons with cerebral palsy and mental retardation, average age of 50, received functional screenings with referrals to AT-EI services as needed (Hammel, Heller & Ying, 1998). Subjects were rated under two conditions: with AT-EI, and without AT-EI (rating done if AT-EI were removed/not present) using the FIM (UDSMR, 1993) and the ICAP (Bruinks et al., 1986) at the time of screenings and an average of 18 months later. Results showed functional improvement or maintenance trends over time with AT-EI, but not without AT-EI (Hammel, Heller & Ying, 1998; Hammel & Heller, 2000).

A four-year study of 109 adults with developmental disabilities who were trying to transition out of nursing homes to the community examined the long term impact of AT-EI on performance of 32 basic and instrumental ADL (Hammel, Lai & Heller, 1999). By four years post, 25% of the subjects had improved performance, 65% maintained status, and 10% declined in function when rated with AT-EI. This compared to 27% experiencing functional declines when not using AT-EI.

Although these studies are limited, the preliminary findings support the beneficial impact of AT-EI in delaying or decreasing the rate of functional decline for aging adults with developmental disabilities, both within the community and nursing home environments. Such findings are especially worth studying within future randomized clinical trials.

Although function was affected by AT-EI, participants and their caregivers repeatedly stated that they felt the solutions given were largely underutilized in everyday activities (Hammel & Heller, 1999). For example, if a wheelchair was broken or could not be used in an inaccessible environment, all other technology attached to it, including communication and daily living technology, also were not used. ADL technology was often misplaced, lost, not set up correctly, or not appropriate given changing needs. More complex, expensive AT systems were used for small amounts of time during the day, citing problems with lack of information on how to integrate the solutions throughout the day across multiple caregivers, especially given high staff turnover rates in sheltered workshops, day programs and group homes. Consumers and staff discussed a need for long term support and training to update systems to reflect the user's changing needs and activities, and to better integrate the AT-EI into everyday routines.

Surveys of people with intellectual disabilities and their caregivers (Wehmeyer, 1995; 1998; Parette & Vanbiervliet, 1992) also support the need for long term AT-EI training and support across functional and community participation activities. In a survey by Benz and Kenmann (1988) of 262 older adults with mental retardation, 92% expressed a desire to engage in educational activities to keep learning new things, and tied this new learning to ability to stay in the community and prevent or delay dependent care placements. Many of these educational activities could involve information technology use, such as the computer and Internet.

In general, adults with developmental disabilities report very limited computer use and a large unmet need (48-79%) for such technology across educational, community living and socialization activities (Parette & Vanbiervliet, 1992; Wehmeyer, 1995, 1998). Computers are used extensively within early intervention and school programs, yet are rarely considered with adults and caregivers who are aging in place. However, websites such as Family Village (see the resources listed at the end of this volume) provide a forum for enabling such use, including easy to use "pen pal" and chat room postings to enable consumers to develop supportive networks with others with similar lifestyles and technology needs. The site also links consumers and caregivers to information about developmental disability and aging, and product sites. Consumers have also developed personal picture-based sites to share their life stories, and self advocacy/leadership development sites, thus demonstrating that computers can be used effectively. AT-EI service providers could assist consumers and caregivers by:

- performing activity analyses to determine how to optimize use of the computer as a tool within everyday activities (educational, social, health and wellness, time management, etc.),
- analyzing the sensorimotor, cognitive and psychosocial skills involved in these activities,
- performing product/activity feature analyses to match consumers and caregivers to appropriate computer hardware, software, activities and websites.

Participation and Environment Findings and Implications

Societal participation and the physical and social environment are so closely linked when considering AT-EI that they are covered together in this section. Wehmeyer's (1995) survey of adults with mental retardation and their families showed that the *most frequently cited barriers* to AT-EI use were funding, information on how to get AT-EI services and products, qualified service providers, long term training, device complexity, and limited product availability specific to people with intellectual or multiple impairments. Parette and VanBiervliet's (1992) found that over 29% paid for AT by themselves or through family, and that very few were offered alternative funding options (e.g., credit plan) or an opportunity to try the AT before buying it. All of these issues reflect societal level barriers to AT-EI use.

A qualitative study of 11 adults with developmental disabilities confirmed these survey results, and explored an additional societal attitudinal barrier (Eidson & Vogtle, 1999). Participants reported problems with using power wheelchairs in the community due to inadequate physical accessibility. However, when forced to use a manual dependent chair, they felt that people treated them as less capable or incompetent. They also reported that the power mobility technology did not allow them to get close to others when socializing, thus the AT that symbolized independence in mobility negatively impacted upon social participation. These findings point to the impact of AT-EI upon perceptions of identity, competence, and life role choices in light of significant, ongoing societal barriers (Gill, 1997; Hammel, 1999).

Other studies have examined differences in acceptance of different types of AT-EI. In a study of AT use with older adults with cognitive impairments primarily due to Alzheimer's Disease, devices to accommodate physical impairments were more readily accepted and used than those for cognitive impairments (e.g., memory aids, schedulers, safety devices); however, people were more satisfied with cognitive devices once used (Nochajski, Tomita & Mann, 1996). This suggests that cognitive aides may take longer to initially accept and learn, however, are seen as beneficial *once they are incorporated into the daily routine* of the person and their caregivers.

A study of AT use among adults with developmental disabilities showed that persons in nursing homes used less AT to address a greater number of functional limitations than those in the community (Mendolson, Heller & Factor, 1995). Thus, living context was directly related to equitable access to AT. Results also showed that people who were living at home with their family, versus in community-based group homes, were more likely to use AT to help the caregiver than to increase the consumer's personal independence. This suggests that there may be a family dynamic in which caregivers might perceive doing a task for the person as more supportive rather than watching them struggle with using AT to do it more independently, or easier than taking the time to set up and maintain the AT-EI. As caregivers age themselves, we can anticipate even greater difficulty in maintaining and supporting AT-EI use over time.

Gerontology theories can provide a framework for better understanding the complex interaction between the person and the environment, especially when considering AT-EI. Lawton's Person/Environment Competence Model (1982) stresses the importance of understanding the *person-environment interaction.* The environment is defined more broadly than physical space to include social, cultural, and societal factors. In order to maintain or increase quality of life and participation during aging, optimal levels of press, in the forms of opportunities/challenges *and* stressors, is needed. Too much press, such as experienced when an environment or way of doing things drastically changes (e.g., moving from walking to a wheelchair or moving from the parent's home to a group or nursing home) can result in behavioral reactions to anxiety and fear, increased rates of AT-EI abandonment, and resulting decreases in activity. Too little press, such as what might be encountered in a nursing home or sheltered workshop with little challenge, can result in boredom, apathy, reduced motivation to participate, and learned helplessness over time.

Corcoran and Gitlin (1992) applied Lawton's Competence Press model within a program targeted toward building the competence of caregivers of older adults with Alzheimer's Disease in the home environment. Interventions centered around identifying functional, behavioral and environmental issues, and problem solving through strategies (including those that could involve AT-EI) with the caregiver/client dyad to prevent or decrease these stressors yet still afford opportunities to function and socialize in the natural home environment. The interventions were delivered in multiple (four), but shorter (1 hour maximum) sessions so caregivers and clients could fully participate and process information from session to session. Results indicated that clients and caregivers both benefited from the program.

Although people with long term intellectual disabilities face different disability and aging issues, they are even more likely to use AT-EI across multiple home and community settings over a longer time period. Such a targeted, theory-based intervention approach could be used within AT-EI interventions and programming to enable the client and their caregivers to develop long term problem solving and coping strategies that can be applied to future life situations.

Qualitative data from caregivers and community agency staff in the study by Hammel and Heller (1999) also support this need for long term support and consumer/caregiver competence building. Beyond delivery of specific AT-EI solutions, consumers and caregivers repeatedly identified the need to assume an *AT user role* to integrate AT within everyday life habits and routines. Essential activities of the AT user role included learning how to set-up, install/program, maintain, repair, troubleshoot, creatively adapt, consistently update, and stay informed about AT-EI. The primary implication for practitioners is that AT-EI interventions need to include both the consumer and their caregivers; focus upon integrating AT-EI into everyday activities, roles and routines; and recommend information resources and social support networks to maintain this integration over time long after the therapist has left the scene.

CONCLUSIONS AND FUTURE RESEARCH IMPLICATIONS

This article summarizes existing and new knowledge about aging with a developmental disability; the impact of AT-EI services and products across impairment, activity and societal participation levels; and implications for AT-EI service deliverers. Grounding AT-EI assessments within activities within everyday contexts offers a way to better assess the person's abilities and capabilities, and the influence of the physical and social environment that often supercedes isolated impairment in the long term. Therapists can systematically adjust components within the environment (e.g., type of AT used, setting, lighting, type or amount of social support) and the activity (e.g., sequence, time of day, number of steps or cues given) to change functional performance. Offering training and practice opportunities across settings and under different conditions (e.g., simulate different problems that may occur with AT-EI over time) rather than repeated practice of the same skill in the same setting can increase the probability of integrating AT-EI into everyday routines.

Interventions that target the consumer, caregivers and staff together in more frequent but shorter opportunities to learn how to use and troubleshoot AT-EI within daily routines, life roles, and environments appear to be effective for people with cognitive impairments, but have not yet been tested for aging adults with developmental disabilities.

Increasing focus on long term resource management (e.g., control over the people, technologies, systems, and information to stay in the community and in control of the AT-EI regardless of level of function or impairment), and development of social support networks also appears to be a significant need within AT-EI service delivery for consumers and caregivers.

Although we have increasing knowledge of impairment, environmental issues such as funding, access to information, quality of services, resources to support AT-EI use in everyday life (e.g., long term training and social support), and societal attitudes about people with developmental disabilities repeatedly emerge as primary barriers to AT-EI use. Given these issues, advocacy for improved later life programming, and future research to justify the need for and impact of AT-EI interventions within these programs, is critical. AT-EI service deliverers can use the research cited throughout this article to justify the AT-EI need and impact within individual interventions; however, advocacy with disability rights and related aging groups also needs to occur to promote increased funding for community-based program development.

Targeted programs to transition people out of dependent care placements, and to support people to live and participate in the community as they age are greatly needed. AT-EI service providers could be key in linking consumers with the technology, environmental adaptations, and resources to support community living. If community living and participation are valued outcomes for all members of society, programs also need to be developed within public settings such as Senior Centers, Centers for Independent Living, and local health and wellness centers which traditionally have not been focused on or responsive to the needs of aging adults with intellectual disabilities and their caregivers. These program development efforts need to include and give voice to people with developmental disabilities who often are not considered during such decisions.

AT-EI can be effective strategies for optimizing health, activity, access and community participation–they can also be effective mechanisms for supporting self and community advocacy across the lifespan. Therapists can play a key role as interface specialists in linking consumers with the most effective AT-EI to support and maintain these outcomes over time.

REFERENCES

Benz, M., & Kennann, K. (1988). Educational experiences, needs, and interests of older adults with mental retardation. *Educational Gerontology, 14*, 509-523.

Bess, F.H., Lichtenstein, M.J., & Logan, S.A. (1991). In: W.F. Rintelmann (ed.) *Hearing Assessment, 2nd Edition.* Austin, TX: PROED.

Bidwell, A. (1999). RRTC focuses on innovation in eye care. *ADDVANTAGE.* Chicago, IL: RRTC on Aging and Mental Retardation.

Braddock, D., Hemp, R., Parish, S., & Westrich, J. (1998). *The State of the States in Developmental Disabilities, 5th Edition.* Washington DC: American Association on Mental Retardation.

Bruinks, R., Hill, B., Weatherman, R., & Woodcock, R. (1986). *Inventory for Client and Agency Planning.* Allen, TX: DLM Teaching Resources.

Carr, J., & Shepard, R. (1992). *A motor relearning programme for stroke.* Rockville, MD: Aspen.

Connolly, B.H. (1998). General effects of aging on persons with developmental disabilities. *Topics in Geriatric Rehabilitation,* 13(3), 1-18.

Corcoran, M., & Gitlin, L. (1992). Dementia management: An occupational therapy home-based intervention for caregivers. *AJOT, 46*(9), 801-808.

Cress, C.J., & Tew, J.P. (1990). Cognitive skills associated with the operation of various computer interfaces. 13th Annual RESNA Conference. Washington DC. 88-89.

Developmental Disabilities Assistance and Bill of Rights Act Amendments of 1994, PL 103-230. (1994). U.S. Congressional Report.

Eidson, C., & Vogtle, L. (1999). *Analysis of the Opinions of Urban Wheelchair Users with Developmental Disabilities Regarding Manual Wheelchair Design.* Unpublished master's thesis. University of Alabama at Birmingham Occupational Therapy Program, Birmingham, AL.

Gill, C. (1997). Four types of integration in disability identity development. *Journal of Vocational Rehabilitation, 9*, 36-46.

Gill, C., & Brown, L. (2000). Overview of health issues of older women with intellectual disabilities. *Physical & Occupational Therapy in Geriatrics, 18*(1), 23-36.

Gitlin L.N., Levine R.E., & Geiger C. (1993). Adaptive device use in the home by older adults with mixed disabilities. *Archives of Physical Medicine and Rehabilitation, 74*, 149-52.

Gitlin L.N.., Schemm R.L., Landsberg L., & Burgh D. (1996). Factors predicting assistive device use in the home by older people following rehabilitation. *Journal of Aging & Health, 8*(4), 554-75.

Hammel, J. (1999). The Life Rope: a transactional approach to exploring worker and life role development. *Work*, 12, 47-60.

Hammel, J., & Heller, T. (2000). *The long-term impact of assistive technology interventions on self management and community living by adults with developmental disabilities.* Manuscript in preparation. University of Illinois at Chicago.

Hammel, J., Heller, T., & Ying, G. (1998). Outcomes of assistive technology services and use by adults with developmental disabilities. *Proceedings of the Rehabilitation Engineering and Assistive Technology Society of North America*, Minneapolis, MN.

Hammel, J., Lai, J. & Heller, T. (1999). Functional and societal participation outcomes of assistive technology and environmental modifications for adults with developmental disabilities. *Proceedings of the Annual Rehabilitation Engineering and Assistive Technology Society of North America Conference,* Long Beach, CA.

Heller, T. (2000). Supporting adults with intellectual disabilities and their families in planning and advocacy: A literature review. *Physical & Occupational Therapy in Geriatrics, 18*(1), 59-73.

Heller, T., & Factor, A. (1998). Research advances and research directions on aging with mental retardation. Chicago, IL: Aging and MR RRTC Clearinghouse, UIC.

Jacobson, J., & Janicki, M. (1983). Observed prevalence of multiple developmental disabilities. *Mental Retardation, 21*(3), 87-94.

Janicki, M.P., & Jacobsen, J.W. (1986). Generational trends in sensory, physical, and behavioral abilities among older mentally retarded persons. *American Journal of Mental Deficiency, 90,* 490-500.

Janicki, M.P., & MacEachron, A.E. (1984). Residential, health and social service needs of elderly developmentally disabled persons. *Gerontologist, 24,* 128-137.

Janicki, M.P., Otis, J.P., Puccio, P.S., Rettig, J.H., & Jacobson, J.W. (1985). Service needs among older developmentally disabled persons. In M.P. Janicki and H.M. Wisniewski (eds). *Aging and Developmental Disabilities, Issues and Approaches.* Baltimore, MD: Paul H. Brookes.

Kielhofner, G., Mallinson, T., Crawford, C., Nowak, M., Rigby, M., Henry, A., & Walens, D. (1998). The Occupational Performance History Interview (OPHI) II. Test Manual. Chicago, IL: University of Illinois at Chicago MOHO Clearinghouse.

Kohlman Thompson, L. (1992). *Kohlman Evaluation of Living Skills (KELS), 3rd Edition.* Bethesda, MD: AOTA.

LaPlante, M., Hendershot, G., & Moss, A. (1992). Assistive technology devices and home accessibility features: Prevalence, payment, needs and trends. *Advance Data, 217.* Washington DC: US Department of Health and Human Services, Centers for Disease Control.

Law, M., Baptiste, S., Carswell, A., McColl, M., Polatajko, H., & Pollock, N. (1994). *Canadian Occupational Performance Measure, 2nd Edition.* Toronto, Ontario: Canadian Association of Occupational Therapists.

Lawton, M.P. (1982). Competence, environmental press and the adaptation of older people. In M. Powell Lawton, P.G. Windley, & T.O. Byerts (Eds.), *Aging and the Environment.* New York: Springer.

Mann, W.C., Ottenbacher, K.J., Fraas, L., Tomita, M., & Granger, C.V. (1999). Effectiveness of assistive technology and environmental interventions in maintaining independence and reducing home care costs for the frail elderly: A randomized controlled trial. *Archives of Family Medicine, 8,* 210-217.

Mazess, R.B. (1987). Bone densiometry in osteoporosis. *Interns and Medical Specialists, 8,* 133.

Mathiowetz & Haugen. (1994). Motor behavior research: Implications for therapeutic approaches to central nervous system dysfunction. *AJOT,* 48(8), 733-745.

McNeil, J.M. (1997). Americans with disabilities: 1994-95. *Current Population Reports,* pp.70-61.

Mendelson, L., Heller, T., & Factor, A. (1995). The transition from nursing homes to community living for people with developmental disabilities: An assessment of the assistive technology needs and usage. *Technology and Disability, 4,* 261-267.

Miller, C.A. (1992). Biophysical development during late adulthood. In C.S. Schuster & S.S. Ashburn (Eds.), *The process of human development: A holistic life-span approach* (3rd. ed., pp. 804-830). Philadelphia: J. P. Lippincott Company.

Nochajski, S. (2000). The impact of age-related changes on the functioning of older adults with developmental disabilities. *Physical & Occupational Therapy in Geriatrics, 18*(1), 5-21.

Nochajski, S., Tomita, M. & Mann, W. (1996). The use and satisfaction with assistive devices by older persons with cognitive impairments: A pilot intervention study. *Topics in Geriatric Rehabilitation, 12*(2), 40-53.

Oliver R., Blathwayt J., Brackley C., & Tamaki T. (1993). Development of the Safety Assessment of Function and the Environment for Rehabilitation (SAFER) tool. *Canadian Journal of Occupational Therapy, 60*(2), 78-82.

Parette, H., & Vanbiervliet, A. (1992). Tentative findings of a study of the technology needs and use patterns of persons with mental retardation. *Journal of Intellectual Disability Research, 36,* 7-27.

Poon, L.W., Gurland, B., Eisdorfer, C., Crook, T., Thompson, L.W., Kaszniak, A., & Davis, K. (eds.). *Handbook for the Clinical Assessment of Older Adults.* Washington DC: APA.

Presperin Pedersen, J. (1995). Wheelchair seating intervention for person with developmental disabilities living in a skilled nursing facility: The "Bogard" consent decree. *Technology and Disability, 4,* 269-273.

Rice, C.L. (1989). Strength in an elderly population. *Archives of Physical Medicine and Rehabilitation, 70,* 391-397.

Russell, J.N., Hendershot, G.E., LeClere, F., Howie, J.H. (1997). Trends and differential use of assistive technology devices: United States, 1994. *Advance Data, 292.* Hyattsville, MD: Center for Disease Control.

Scherer M.J. (1991). The Matching Person & Technology (MPT) Model and assessment instruments. Rochester, NY: Author.

Seltzer, G.B., & Luchterhand, C. (1994). Health and well-being of older persons with developmental disabilities: a clinical review. In: M.M. Seltzer, M.W. Krause, & M.P. Janicki (eds.) *Life course perspectives on adulthood and old age.* Washington DC: American Association on Mental Retardation.

Trieschmann, R.B. (1987). *Aging with a disability.* New York: Demos.

Uniform Data Set for Medical Rehabilitation (1993). *A Guide for the Uniform Data Set for Medical Rehabilitation (Adult FIM), version 4.0.* Buffalo, NY: SUNY-Buffalo.

Walz, T., Harper, D., & Wilson, J. (1986). The aging developmental disabled person: A review. *Gerontologist, 26,* 622-629.

Wehmeyer, M. (1995). The use of assistive technology by people with mental retardation and barriers to this outcome: A pilot study. *Technology and Disability, 4,* 195-204.

Wehmeyer, M. (1998). National survey of the use of assistive technology by adults with mental retardation. *Mental Retardation, 36*, (1), 44-51.

WHO (2000). *ICIDH-2: International Classification of Functioning and Disability.* Website address: http://www.who.int/icidh/index.htm (1/20/2000). Geneva: World Health Organization.

Whiteneck G.G., Charlifue S.W., Gerhart K.A., Overholser J.D., Richardson G.N. (1992). Quantifying Handicap: A New Measure of Long Term Rehabilitation Outcomes. *Archives of Physical Medicine and Rehabilitation, 73*, 519-526.

Supporting Adults with Intellectual Disabilities and Their Families in Planning and Advocacy: A Literature Review

Tamar Heller, PhD

SUMMARY. This paper reviews the literature on later-life planning interventions that aim to support adults with intellectual disabilities and their families in planning and advocacy. While most of these interventions include both the person with a disability and the families at least to some degree, they differ in terms of the target group that is the primary focus. Hence, this review first examines family-focused strategies and secondly strategies focused on the person with disabilities. Thirdly, the paper discusses implications for further practice and research on promoting planning for the future of adults with intellectual disabilities. *[Article copies available for a fee from The Haworth Document Delivery Service: 1-800-342-9678. E-mail address: <getinfo@haworthpressinc.com> Website: <http://www.HaworthPress.com>]*

Tamar Heller is Professor and Director of the Rehabilitation Research and Training Center on Aging with Mental Retardation, Department of Disability and Human Development, University of Illinois at Chicago, 1640 West Roosevelt Road, Chicago, IL 60608.

Preparation of this article was supported in part by funding from the Rehabilitation Research and Training Center on Aging with Mental Retardation, University of Illinois at Chicago, through the U.S. Department of Education, National Institute on Disability and Rehabilitation Research, Grant No. H133B980046. The opinions contained in this publication are those of the grantee and do not necessarily reflect those of the U.S. Department of Education.

[Haworth co-indexing entry note]: "Supporting Adults with Intellectual Disabilities and Their Families in Planning and Advocacy: A Literature Review." Heller, Tamar. Co-published simultaneously in *Physical & Occupational Therapy in Geriatrics* (The Haworth Press, Inc.) Vol. 18, No. 1, 2000, pp. 59-73; and: *Aging and Developmental Disability: Current Research, Programming, and Practice Implications* (ed: Joy Hammel, and Susan M. Nochajski) The Haworth Press, Inc., 2000, pp. 59-73. Single or multiple copies of this article are available for a fee from The Haworth Document Delivery Service [1-800-342-9678, 9:00 a.m. - 5:00 p.m. (EST). E-mail address: getinfo@haworthpressinc.com].

KEYWORDS. Mental retardation, intellectual disabilities, future planning, families, self-determination

While planning for the future is a task faced by all persons as they age, the need for adults with intellectual disabilities and their families to conduct later-life planning has been well-documented (Heller & Factor, 1993; Freedman, Krauss, & Seltzer, 1997). Over 60% of persons with intellectual disabilities live with family caregivers (Fujiura, 1998), of which 25% are 60 years and older (Braddock, 1999). Both family caregivers and the adult with disabilities face age-related changes, including declining health, changing roles, and retirement issues. Without adequate plans in place, these adults often face the prospect of emergency placements in inappropriate settings, inadequate financial plans, difficulties for siblings and other relatives, and disruptive transitions after families can no longer provide care. When families do seek residential placements they confront long waiting lists, with 83,101 people with intellectual disabilities on waiting lists for residential services nationally (Prouty & Lakin, 1998).

Many parents do not discuss future plans with other family members or with their son or daughter with disabilities (Heller & Factor, 1994; Smith & Tobin, 1989). There is a growing recognition that people with intellectual disabilities need to be active participants in the planning process and that they can often make competent decisions about their lives. However, many of these adults have had little experience not only in making long term plans, but also in making choices in their daily lives (Heller, Factor, Sterns, & Sutton, 1996; Lakin, Burwell, Hayden, & Jackson, 1992; Sands & Kuzleski, 1994). Furthermore, persons with intellectual disabilities are often unaware of how their lives may change as they age with regard to their health, work, leisure, and living arrangements.

This paper reviews the literature on later-life planning interventions that aim to support adults with intellectual disabilities and their families in future planning and advocacy. While most of these interventions include both the person with a disability and the family to some degree, they differ with respect to the target group that is the primary focus. Hence, this review first examines family-focused strategies and secondly, strategies focused on the person with disabilities. Thirdly, the paper discusses implications for practice and research on promoting planning for the future.

FAMILY ISSUES AND INTERVENTIONS

Planning Needs

Key aspects which usually need to be addressed by families in planning for their relative include future living arrangements, guardianship and other less restrictive alternatives, financial planning, advanced directives in health care, and general lifestyle choices. Planning for future living arrangements of a family member with disabilities is often anxiety-provoking as it reminds families of their mortality. Also, it can remind families of concerns regarding family responsibility, separation, and independence (Freedman et al., 1997). Furthermore, parents who have provided life-long care for their child may be reluctant to relinquish their role. Research findings indicate that between 25% and 50% of families have made plans for their son's or daughter's future living arrangement; and nearly half want the child to live with another family member (Heller & Factor, 1994). The degree to which families make residential plans depend on socio-economic resources, personal coping styles, and the type of options available in their communities (Heller & Factor, 1991; Freedman et al., 1997). Often, families from minority racial/ethnic backgrounds are less tied into the service system and are less likely to have made plans for the future care of their relative than non-Hispanic Whites (Heller & Factor, 1994; McCallion, Janicki, & Grant-Griffin, 1997).

Legal and financial planning are additional challenges for families who want to assure financial resources for their relative without losing government benefits and who want to obtain guardianship if their relative is deemed incompetent. Heller and Factor (1991) found that nearly two-thirds of families caring for members with intellectual disabilities age 30 years and older had made financial plans and nearly one-quarter had made guardianship plans. However, families and professionals often lacked adequate legal and financial information resulting in plans that did not protect government benefits or that needlessly deprived adults with intellectual disabilities of their rights.

Numerous assessments of families' service needs have noted that the highest unmet needs were for information regarding residential programs, financial plans, and guardianship. Also, they have major needs for case management, advocacy, and support groups (Heller & Factor, 1994; Kelly & Kropf, 1995). One source of information for families is psycho-educational groups. These groups are typically led by professionals or by families who have been through the planning process. They can provide not only information on service options and coping strategies, but also can provide psychological support. Smith, Majeski and McClenny (1996) found that caregivers of adults with intellectual disabilities who participated in such groups reported that they benefited from the information on future planning and service options, and from opportunities to interact with other parents having similar concerns.

Future Planning Program Approaches

In the literature there are examples of several model projects in the United States and Canada that have sought to provide information and encouragement to families in making long term plans for their adult family member with a disability. Examples include the Family Futures Planning Project in Rhode Island (Susa & Clark, 1996), Planned Lifetime Advocacy Network in British Columbia (PLAN) (Etmanski, 1997), Family-to-Family Project in Massachusetts (*Community Services Reporter*, 1999; Griffiths, 1997) and Rehabilitation Research and Training Center (RRTC) on Aging with Mental Retardation Multicultural Family Future Planning Project (Preston & Heller, 1996). Each project differed in terms of the families targeted, the curriculum and information provided, and the way support was provided. While these programs primarily targeted families of persons with intellectual disabilities, some also included families of persons with other disabilities (e.g., PLAN and the Multicultural Family Future Planning Project). This list of programs exemplifies model programs for which there is written literature and which focus on long term planning with older caregivers. There are many other programs that address future planning of younger families coping with transition of their child with disabilities from adolescence to adulthood (e.g., Wehmeyer & Kelchner, 1995) or more general person-centered planning approaches (e.g., Pearpoint, Forest, & O'Brien, 1996).

The Family Futures Planning Project in Rhode Island targeted older family caregivers (Susa & Clark, 1996). The 10-session curriculum included information on such topics as housing options, estate planning, and home and community based services. Also, some sessions dealt directly with issues of the aging caregiver, their emotional and physical health, and leisure activities. A paid facilitator assisted families with developing a plan and building a support network. The focus was on the family's needs rather than on the needs of the individual with an intellectual disability. The aging and developmental disabilities systems successfully collaborated in supporting families through the project. Only 18 families participated; however, due to the intimacy of the small groups, families were able to share experiences and support one another. As part of this project families identified barriers to future planning and began to move ahead in the process of making change leading to future planning.

The Planned Lifetime Advocacy Network (PLAN) in British Columbia, Canada is a family operated non-profit organization (Etmanski, 1997). PLAN receives no government funding, but half of the funding comes directly from families so the scope of families reached is limited to those who can afford membership. PLAN has developed a six step guide to developing a personal future plan: clarifying your vision, building relationships, controlling the home environment, preparing for decision making, developing your will and estate plan, and securing your plan. PLAN provides many levels of support and services and uses mentor families, who attend meetings and visit other families, in addition to paid facilitators that assist with developing a support network. Workshops and technical assistance are provided to families. PLAN also conducts systems advocacy by lobbying at the governmental level. The mission of PLAN is to provide a "lifetime commitment" to families and assist them with creating a secure future for their family member with a disability.

The Family-to-Family Project in Massachusetts targeted all families with a member on the waiting list for residential services (Griffiths, 1997; *Community Services Reporter*, 1999). The project developed eight Family-to-Family Support Centers across the state. Each center's activities varied. Some centers included presentations on special needs trusts and wills, home ownership and consumer controlled housing, circles of support, and self-advocacy. One center compiled a resource manual with information concerning funding sources, housing options, and legal issues and translated it into several languages. Most of the sites conducted outreach to unserved families. Monthly parent support groups were formed where participants shared and exchanged information. Written letters by families and a state survey conducted by the project were sent to legislators to address systems advocacy.

The RRTC Multicultural Family Future Planning project (Preston & Heller, 1996) conducted legal and financial training with 220 families at 17 sites. One site included primarily African-American families and another site targeted Hispanic families. The training of family and staff members comprised two-day training workshops conducted by a lawyer and parent of an adult with intellectual disabilities. In addition case coordinators received training on ways to provide support and follow-up to families.

Although most of these interventions did not report empirical results, anecdotal information suggests limited success of these projects in stimulating future planning. The key initiatives have generally included a training component, but varied as to whether they used paid facilitators or other parents as mentors. None of the key projects included peer mentors or training for the person with intellectual disabilities.

While families generally note a high need for training on futures planning and rate such training very positively, they often do not follow-up the training with concrete actions or plans. The Planned Advocacy and Network Project noted that only 5% of families who attended their training workshops made plans (Etmanski, 1996). Similarly, six months after the RRTC legal and financial training most families still had not made much progress in developing plans (Preston & Heller, 1996). Their preliminary survey of families who participated in the training indicated that most families expressed intentions to plan but felt that they needed more support in dealing with the psychological issues and in negotiating the service system. Yet, they rated these workshops very positively.

The Family Futures Project in Rhode Island (Susa & Clark, 1996) that included training and a paid service facilitator, reported that very few families made plans during the project's 18 month period, but that the project was successful in getting them to progress in the planning process. The PLAN project that included training with family mentoring and ongoing support, reported more success among families who sought ongoing support from other families. The Massachusetts Family-to-Family initiative succeeded in establishing eight family networking centers around the state. Through peer networking these centers enabled families on the waiting list for residential services to learn about ways to develop family-financed housing approaches and advocate for systems change. However, there was no data reported on the degree to which families made futures plans.

In summary, the model family future planning projects found in the literature have not helped families begin to make plans for their relative with intellectual disabilities. However, there have been no empirical evaluations documenting that families have indeed made plans. This type of evaluation would require a long term longitudinal evaluation and planning is a long term process for families that involves not only the parents but also other members of the family and the person with the disability.

LATER-LIFE PLANNING FOR ADULTS WITH INTELLECTUAL DISABILITIES

Later-Life Planning Needs

Many adults with intellectual disabilities lack awareness about making choices and later life issues. This includes awareness of work and retirement options, health and wellness needs, residential living arrangements, and leisure/recreation activities (Sterns, Kennedy, Sed, & Heller, in press). Given the limited work opportunities for adults with intellectual disabilities, with only 26% employed, and the majority employed in sheltered workshops (Yamaki, 1999), retirement has a different meaning than that for the general population. Retirement is rarely discussed with adults having an intellectual disability. In a survey conducted in Ohio addressing retirement programs for older adults with intellectual disabilities (Sutton et al., 1993), retirement planning was very limited, consisting primarily of staff making transition plans based on observing increased fatigue, health changes, and less interest in work. The preferences of the person with a disability were rarely considered in making these transitions.

With regard to health, adults with intellectual disabilities face similar age-related changes as the general population, although there are some subpopulations that experience earlier age-related declines. These include adults with Down syndrome, cerebral palsy, and severe intellectual disabilities (reviewed in Heller, 1997). Adults with intellectual disabilities also have a greater risk of developing secondary conditions partially due to poor health habits and sedentary lifestyles. In particular, they are more vulnerable to obesity and high cholesterol (Rimmer, Braddock, & Marks, 1995). Often these adults have little concept of physical changes that occur with aging or of the consequences of their health behaviors (Heller et al., 1996).

Another key area that needs to be addressed in later-life planning is leisure and recreational activities. As persons decrease their work, leisure activities may take on greater importance. Rogers, Hawkins, and Eklund (1998) report that older adults with intellectual disabilities tend to have few choices in their leisure activities and express dissatisfaction with the leisure activities offered them. However, when they do have more opportunities to participate in their preferred leisure activities, their life satisfaction increases (Hawkins & McClean, 1993).

Later-Life Planning Program Approaches

Later-life planning training aims to increase the knowledge and skills older adults with intellectual disabilities have about later-life issues and to provide opportunities for them to make choices regarding their own lives. Training also focuses on a planning process for making current and future lifestyle changes.

Several training programs have been developed to address various aspects of later-life planning for adults with intellectual disabilities. Laughlin and Cotton's (1994) pre-retirement program (Pre-Retirement Assessment and Planning for Older Adults with Mental Retardation) primarily targeted adults moving from institutional settings to community settings. It includes a planning process for identifying wants and needs, developing plans to achieve them, acting on them, and continually revising those plans as knowledge and experience is gained. It also involves training focused on the changes retirement can bring in work, social roles, support systems, health needs, finances, living arrangements and community involvement. Laughlin and Cotton's (1994) evaluation of the impact of this training on 75 adults with mild to moderate intellectual disabilities (aged 50-72 years) indicated that the training program was effective in teaching the participants about options available during their retirement years. However, the program did not seem to change their attitudes to retirement or their life satisfaction.

Isfeld and Mahon (1997) developed a more narrowly focused intervention that specifically targeted leisure activities: The Later-Life Planning Program. It was modeled after the Supported Leisure Program (Mahon & Martens, 1996) that combines leisure education with a personal futures planning process. Mount and Zwernick (1990) describe Personal Futures Planning as a process for helping people create a life of meaning for the person who is the focus of the planning. Individuals are encouraged to dream about possible futures and to work backwards to develop manageable steps that can lead them to their desired future. This type of planning places the individual with a disability in the position to direct decisions affecting his or her own life.

Incorporating both the leisure education and personal futures planning approaches, the Later-Life Planning Program includes three phases; (a) retirement and leisure awareness and decision-making, (b) PATH planning (Planning Alternative Future for Tomorrow with Hope) (Pearpoint, O'Brien, & Forest, 1993), and (c) leisure initiation. In a study evaluating the impact of this planning process on older adults with intellectual disabilities Mahon and Goatcher (1999) found that this program resulted in higher leisure and life satisfaction for the participants in comparison with the control group. It also resulted in lifestyle changes for many of these adults including full or partial retirement, changes in work assignments, and participation in leisure activities. However, this study included a very small sample of 10 participants in the intervention and 10 control group members.

A more broadly focused later-life planning program is the Person-Centered Planning for Later-Life Curriculum for Persons with Mental Retardation (Sutton, Heller, Sterns, Factor, & Miklos, 1993). Its curriculum teaches adults with intellectual disabilities about current and potential living arrangements, work and retirement options, health and wellness, leisure and recreation activities, use of informal and formal supports. Within these content areas, the participants learn about making choices, setting goals, and making action plans. Also, the curriculum includes a training component for families and staff who provide support to the person with intellectual disabilities. This training teaches the families and staff about later-life options for adults with intellectual disabilities and on ways to support them in making choices and in attaining goals.

This training program incorporates both a lifespan developmental orientation and a person-centered perspective. A lifespan developmental orientation assumes that people can learn new skills and behaviors and are open to change throughout their lives (Baltes & Graf, 1996). Hence, the program aims to increase the awareness and knowledge of adults with intellectual disabilities about later life options and to develop new opportunities for them.

Similarly to the Isfeld and Mahon (1997) Later-Life Planning Program, this training incorporates a person-centered approach (Mount &

Zwernik, 1990). Hence, in addition to teaching skills and knowledge, it helps promote self-determination and quality of life through a planning process incorporating the preferences of the person with intellectual disabilities. It also involves collaboration with people who know the individuals and can support them in achieving their vision. In this training each participant chooses a support person who attends initial staff and family member training and jointly attends two of the 17 training sessions for the adult with disabilities. These support persons are guided to support persons in making choices and in setting and attaining goals. This is encouraged through sharing of assignments with their support person and through joint action planning among the individual with intellectual disabilities, staff, and family members. Another unique aspect of this training program is that it uses peer trainers, persons with intellectual disabilities, as co-trainers. Bandura (1986) has noted the importance of observational learning and peer modeling in teaching people new skills. Peer co-trainers have been effective in teaching adults with intellectual disabilities to make life choices and to learn about service options (Heller & Nelis, 1996).

This training program has been empirically evaluated in two U.S. states, the Netherlands, and Germany. The first study (Heller et al., 1996), conducted in Ohio and Illinois, included 80 older adults with moderate to mild intellectual disabilities (42 in the intervention group and 38 in the comparison group). Participation in the intervention resulted in increased knowledge of later life options in a six-month follow-up. Secondly, the training resulted in increased leisure activity participation for participants who lived with family. The training also resulted in changes in the planning process used by agencies: (a) the preferences of the person with a disability were more likely to be incorporated in the planning process, (b) family members were more likely to attend planning sessions, and (c) agency staff were more likely to encourage the person with a disability to speak up at planning sessions. One unintended consequence of the training was a decrease in life satisfaction for the intervention group in the six-month follow-up. It seemed that increased awareness of options and of ways to increase choice-making also resulted in greater dissatisfaction, particularly with the residential environment.

In order to assess the effectiveness of this curriculum in other countries, the training intervention and research was replicated in Germany and the Netherlands with 75 and 82 intervention participants, respectively. The follow-ups were conducted both at the six month and at the ten month periods. At the ten month assessments the training participants retained the knowledge they had gained on later-life options and had a decrease in life satisfaction (Havemen, 1998).

Following the first evaluation of the Person-Centered Planning for Later-Life Curriculum for Persons with Mental Retardation, it was revised to increase the generalization of choice-making skills and the attainment of goals. This included greater use of role-plays in the training, more assignments for participants to make choices in their natural settings, greater emphasis on working with support persons to help facilitate desired goals. A study of 60 older adults with intellectual disabilities (38 in the intervention group and 22 in the comparison group) evaluating the outcomes of this revised curriculum indicated that it was successful in teaching knowledge of later-life options and choice-making. Participants also made more choices over time than the control group. Unlike the previous study there were no significant changes in life satisfaction for the intervention group. This might be due to the fact that the vast majority of participants (87%) met or partially met their personal goals within ten months after the training. This study also identified the types of supports participants experienced in meeting their goals. Staff persons provided most of the support, e.g., accompanying them to activities, organizing activities, making arrangements with another agency or organization, and providing emotional encouragement to meet goals. Family members provided support by accompanying their relative to activities and by buying needed supplies. Other sources of support for meeting goals included adequate transportation and support from peers or community members.

Although the later-life planning training programs have included families in the process, they have not focused on helping families make plans for the future. Rather, they have tended to focus on more short-term choices and goals and have not adequately addressed issues of future financial and legal arrangements and planning for the time when families can no longer provide caregiving. Hence, by combining both the approaches focusing on families and those focusing on the adult with disabilities, planning can be addressed more comprehensively and is more likely to result in having plans that meet the families' needs.

IMPLICATIONS FOR RESEARCH AND PRACTICE

The planning approaches reviewed in this article have demonstrated effective means to help families learn about future planning issues and to help persons with intellectual disabilities learn about later-life options. However, most of the approaches have had limited success in helping families actually make plans. The projects directed at families primarily tended to neglect training the person with intellectual disabilities, despite the importance of meaningfully including the person with a disability in the planning process. On the other hand, the projects focused on training adults with intellectual disabilities tended to neglect the longer-term future planning issues necessitating greater family input.

Future interventions would benefit from a more comprehensive approach that incorporates both types of training and planning processes. This would include the following aspects: (1) psycho-educational training regarding futures planning for families, (2) training for the person with a disability and support staff, (3) paid facilitator to help families make plans and to provide follow-up consultations, (4) mentoring by other parents and persons with intellectual disabilities who have already gone through the planning process, and (5) networking of families to help promote advocacy and systems change.

The goals of this type of program would be to: (a) increase families' progress in developing future plans, (b) increase the involvement of the family members with intellectual disabilities and siblings in the planning process, (c) reduce family caregiving burden, (d) increase family caregiving satisfaction (e) increase community involvement for individual with intellectual disabilities, (f) decrease dependence on state funding and initiatives for housing crisis, (g) increase tolerance and respect among families, professionals and the person with a disability, and (h) empower individuals to have choice and control in their future plans.

While there are many projects conducting future planning, there is a need to conduct research that: (a) identifies, develops and analyzes best practices and training materials in Futures Planning for adults with intellectual disabilities and their families; (b) describes facilitators and barriers for families in making future plans; and (c) tests the effectiveness of peer training and support interventions on the participation of families and persons with intellectual disabilities in futures planning, knowledge and attitudes towards futures planning, and on caregiving appraisal (burden and satisfaction) of family caregivers.

REFERENCES

Bandura, A. (1986). *Social foundations of thought and action: A social cognitive theory.* Englewood Cliffs, NJ: Prentice Hall.

Braddock, D. (1999). Aging and developmental disabilities: Demographic and policy issues affecting American families. *Mental Retardation, 37,* 155-161.

Community Services Reporter (1999). Family-to-Family project helps to reduce Massachusetts' waiting list. *Community Services Reporter, May 1999,* pp. 4-5.

Etmanski, A. (1996). *Safe and secure: Six steps to creating a personal future plan for people with disabilities.* Burnaby, British Columbia Planned Lifetime Advocacy Network.

Freedman, R. I., Krauss, M. W., & Seltzer, M. M. (1997). Aging parents' residential plans for adults children with mental retardation. *Mental Retardation, 35,* 114-123.

Fujiura, G. T. (1998). Demography of family households. *American Journal on Mental Retardation, 103,* 225-235.

Griffiths, D. (1997). *Waiting in the wings: Full report on a survey of caregivers with family members on the waiting list for residential services from the Massachusetts Department of Mental Retardation.* Waltham, Massachusetts: Family to Family. Technical support provided by the Starr Center for Mental Retardation, Heller Graduate School, Brandeis University.

Haveman, M. (1998, July). *Person-centered planning for later life: An evaluative study of a curriculum for adults with intellectual disability.* Paper presented at the Beit Issie Shapiro Second International Conference on Developmental Disabilities in the Community: Policy, Practice and Research. Jerusalem, Israel.

Hawkins, B. A., & McClean, D. (1993). Delivering services to a diverse aging population: Challenges for the future. *Journal of Health, Physical Education, Recreation, and Dance, 64,* 31-34.

Heller, T. (1997). Aging in persons with mental retardation and their families. In N.Bray (Ed.). *International review of research in mental retardation, vol. 20.* (pp. 99-136) New-York: Academic Press.

Heller, T., & Factor, A. (1991). Permanency planning for adults with mental retardation living with family caregivers. *American Journal of Mental Retardation, 96,* 163-176.

Heller, T., & Factor, A. (1993). Support systems, well-being, and placement decision-making among older parents and their adult children with developmental disabilities. In E. Sutton, A. Factor, B. Hawkins, T. Heller, & G. Seltzer (Eds.), *Older adults with developmental disabilities: Optimizing choice and change* (pp. 107-122). Baltimore: Paul H. Brookes Pub. Co.

Heller, T., & Factor, A. (1994). Facilitating future planning and transitions out of the home. In M.M. Seltzer, M.W. Krauss, & M. Janicki (Eds.), *Life-course perspectives on adulthood and old age.* (pp 39-50). Washington, DC: American Association on Mental Retardation Monograph Series.

Heller, T., & Nelis, T. (1996, May). *Research, training and leadership partnerships: Professionals and self-advocates working together.* Paper presented at the Annual Meeting of the American Association on Mental Retardation, San Antonio, TX.

Heller, T., Sterns, H., Sutton, E., & Factor, A. (1996). Impact of person-centered later life planning training program for older adults with mental retardation. *Journal of Rehabilitation*, 62, 77-83.

Isfeld, C., & Mahon, M. J. (1997). Exploring later life options with older adults with mental retardation: Facilitators manual. Winnipeg, MB: Sturgeon Creek Enterprises, Inc.

Kelly, T. B., & Kropf, N. P. (1995). Stigmatized and perpetual parents: Older parents caring for adult children with lifelong disabilities. *Journal of Gerontological Social Work*, 24, 3-16.

Lakin, K. C., Buwell, B., Hayden, M., & Jackson, M. (1992). *An independent assessment of Minnesota's Medicaid Home and Community Based Services Waiver Program (Report No. 37)*. Minneapolis: University of Minnesota, Center for Residential Services and Community Living, Institute on Community Integration.

Laughlin, C. & Cotten, P. D. (1994). Efficacy of a pre-retirement planning intervention for aging individuals with mental retardation. *Journal of Intellectual Disability Research*, 38, 317-328.

Mahon, M. J. & Martens, C. (1996). Planning for the future: The impact of leisure education for adults with developmental disabilities in supported employment settings. *Journal of Applied Recreation Research*, 21, 283-312.

Mahon, M. J., & Goatcher, S. (1999) Later-life planning for older adults with mental retardation: A field experiment. *Mental Retardation*, 37, 371-382.

McCallion, P., Janicki, M., & Grant-Griffin, L. (1997). Exploring the impact of culture and acculturation on older families caregiving for persons with developmental disabilities. *Family Relations*, 46, 347-358.

Mount, B., & Zwernick, K. (1990) Making futures happen: A manual for facilitators of personal futures planning. St. Paul, MN: Metropolitan Council.

Pearpoint, J., Forest, M., & O'Brien, J. (1996). Circles of friends and PATH: Powerful tools to help build caring communities. In S. B. Stainback, & W. C. Stainback (Eds.). *Inclusion: A guide for educators* (pp. 67-86). Baltimore, MD: Paul H. Brookes Publishing Co.

Preston, L., & Heller, T. (1996, October). *Working partnerships to individualize future planning for older families from diverse groups*. Paper presented at the Sixth Lexington Conference on Aging and Developmental Disabilities. Lexington, KY.

Prouty, R., & Lakin, K. C. (Eds.). (1998). *Residential services for persons with developmental disabilities: Status and trends through 1997*. Minneapolis, MN: University of Minnesota, Research and Training Center on Community Living, Institute on Community Integration.

Rimmer, J., Braddock, D., & Marks, B. (1995). Health characteristics and behaviors of adults with mental retardation mental retardation residing in three living arrangements. *Research in Developmental Disabilities*, 16, 489-499.

Rogers, N. B., Hawkins, B. A., & Eklund, S. J. (1998). The nature of leisure in the lives of older adults with intellectual disability. *Journal of Intellectual Disability Research*, 42, 122-130.

Sands, D. J., & Kozleski, E. B. (1994). Quality of life difference between adults with and without disabilities. *Education and Training in Mental Retardation and Developmental Disabilities*, 29, 90-101.

Smith, G., Majeski, R. & McClenny, B. (1996). Psychoeducational support groups for aging parents: Development and preliminary outcomes. *Mental Retardation, 34,* 172-181.

Smith, G. & Tobin, S. (1989). Permanency planning among older parents of adults with lifelong disabilities. *Journal of Gerontological Social Work, 14,* 35-59.

Sterns, H. L., Kennedy, H. E.., Sed, C., & Heller, T. (in press). Later-life planning and retirement. In M. P. Janicki & E. F. Ansello (Eds.). *Community support for aging: Adults with lifelong disabilities.* Baltimore: Paul H. Brookes.

Susa, C. & Clark, P. (1996). *Drafting a blueprint for change: The coordinators manual.* Kingston, Rhode Island: University of Rhode Island.

Sutton, E., Heller, T., Sterns, H. L., Factor, A., & Miklos, S. (1993). *Person-Centered Planning for later life: A curriculum for adults with mental retardation.* Akron, Ohio: Rehabilitation Research and Training Center on Aging with mental retardation; the University of Illinois at Chicago and the University of Akron.

Sutton, E., Sterns, H., & Schwartz, L. (1993). Realities of retirement and pre-retirement planning. In E. Sutton, A. Factor, B. Hawkins, T. Heller, & G. Seltzer (Eds.), *Older adults with developmental disabilities: Optimizing choice and change* (pp. 95-106). Baltimore: Paul H. Brookes Pub. Co.

Wehmeyer, M. L. & Kelchner, K. (1995). *Whose future is it anyway? A student-directed transition planning process.* Boston, MA: Women's Educational Equity Act Publishing Center.

Yamaki, K. (1999). Employment and income status of adults with developmental disabilities living in the community. *Doctoral thesis.* Chicago: University of Illinois at Chicago.

Challenges to Aging in Place:
The Elder Adult with MR/DD

Joseph E. Campbell, OTR/L
E. Adel Herge, MS, OTR/L

SUMMARY. The growing population of elder adults in the United States include those diagnosed with MR/DD. Their presence in the community results from governmental policy changes, leading to community based health and residential services. This article will focus on the challenges facing the elder adult with MR/DD "aging in place." Perspectives of care for persons with MR/DD, both historical and contemporary, will be reviewed. Challenges that are experienced by this population, their families and the service community are described and the role of occupational and physical therapists in assisting the elder adult to "age in place" in the community is presented. *[Article copies available for a fee from The Haworth Document Delivery Service: 1-800-342-9678. E-mail address: <getinfo@haworthpressinc.com> Website: <http://www.HaworthPress.com>]*

KEYWORDS. Elder adult, MR/DD, aging in place, therapy

INTRODUCTION TO THE POPULATION

Aging of the American population is reflected in the 1990 U.S. Census which reported there are 33 million people age 65 years or

Joseph E. Campbell is Senior Occupational Therapist, Woods Services, Route 213, Langhorne, PA 19047. E. Adel Herge is Instructor, Department of Occupational Therapy, Thomas Jefferson University, 130 South 9th Street, Suite 820, Philadelphia, PA 19107.

[Haworth co-indexing entry note]: "Challenges to Aging in Place: The Elder Adult with MR/DD." Campbell, Joseph E., and E. Adel Herge. Co-published simultaneously in *Physical & Occupational Therapy in Geriatrics* (The Haworth Press, Inc.) Vol. 18, No. 1, 2000, pp. 75-90; and: *Aging and Developmental Disability: Current Research, Programming, and Practice Implications* (ed: Joy Hammel, and Susan M. Nochajski) The Haworth Press, Inc., 2000, pp. 75-90. Single or multiple copies of this article are available for a fee from The Haworth Document Delivery Service [1-800-342-9678, 9:00 a.m. - 5:00 p.m. (EST). E-mail address: getinfo@haworthpressinc.com].

older (Bonder & Wagner, 1994). This includes individuals diagnosed with mental retardation and developmental disabilities. This segment of the aging population appears to be increasing in numbers for a variety of reasons.

First, the aging process is believed to begin earlier in individuals with mental retardation/developmental disability (MR/DD). Some researchers maintain that the aging process begins at age 55 for persons with mental retardation (Seltzer & Seltzer, 1985). Secondly, advances in medical technology and health care have helped to increase the longevity of persons with MR/DD. For instance, persons with Down Syndrome had a life expectancy of less than 10 years old in 1929, but with advances in cardiac care and surgical procedures the life expectancy of these persons are beginning to mirror that of the non-disabled population (Chicoine & McGuire, 1997; Connolly, 1998). Lastly, this population has become more visible in the general community. Elder adults with MR/DD are increasingly using community health care systems to address medical issues associated with aging as well as those conditions associated with specific syndromes.

Individuals with MR/DD often experience a need for additional support in daily activities due to physiological and psychological changes associated with aging. Chronic health problems similar to those experienced in the general population have been identified in elder adults with MR/DD (Anderson, 1993; Kapell, Nightingale, Rodriquez, Lee, Zigman, & Schupf, 1998). These include arthritis, hypertension, osteoporosis, hip fractures, cerebral vascular accidents (CVA), and cardiac anomalies. However, the population of adults with MR/DD may have a higher incidence of specific disabilities associated with their primary diagnoses and syndromes. For example, Kapell et al. (1998) reported a high incidence of thyroid disorders, nonischemic heart disorders and visual impairments associated with Down Syndrome. Beange, McElduff and Baker (1995) found that elders with mental retardation have increased risk factors for cardiovascular disease as well as a higher number of chronic diseases with increased morbidity and mortality rates compared to the general public.

There are also psychological issues related to aging. The elder adult with MR/DD may be experiencing emotional disorders, anxiety, phobias and depression (Foelker & Luke, 1989; Rojahn, Warren & Ohringer, 1994). These can result from physiological changes, long term pharmaceutical use or changes in living situation or lifestyle (DiGiovanni, 1978; Foelker & Luke, 1989). The elder adult with mental retardation is also at risk for dementia (Foelker & Luke, 1989). Lastly, individuals with MR/DD often have led sedentary lifestyles which may be complicated by eating a diet high in sugar, fat and cholesterol and perhaps, excessive use of caffeine and tobacco (Edgerton, Gaston, Kelly & Ward, 1994).

Along with changes in health status, the adult with MR/DD may experience changes within family and living arrangements. Family caregivers are also encountering the health and social changes that accompany the aging process–decreased stamina and energy, increased use of health care resources, changes in financial status and changes in family constellation with illness and death of spouses (Bonder & Wagner, 1994; Janicki, 1992). These families may be connecting with support systems for their aging relative with DD, for themselves and/or for other family members, after 50-60 years of privately caring for their family member. This reliance on social support systems may be new, and the unfamiliar systems can be unfamiliar overwhelming for families. Likewise, social support systems may become overwhelmed by the complex needs of these families who are entering the system "late in the game" (Herge & Campbell, 1999).

This article will focus on the concept of the elder adult with MR/DD aging in place, that is, growing old in a familiar environment (Rowles, 1993). Historical and contemporary perspectives of care for persons with MR/DD will be reviewed. The challenges that are experienced by this population, their families and the service community are described and the role of the occupational and physical therapist in assisting the elder MR/DD adult to age in place in the community is presented. Several case examples illustrating challenges and opportunities experienced by the authors working with elder adults in group homes are presented.

HISTORICAL AND CURRENT PERSPECTIVES OF CARE

At the turn of the 20th century, persons with MR/DD had limited housing options, particularly if they were from poor or low-income families. Options included living in poorhouses, hospitals or at home. Other persons, generally those from more affluent families, were placed in small private residential schools (Ferguson, 1994). Medical, nursing and therapeutic services were typically provided on site and these were regarded as limited in quality (Wolfensberger, 1991). Later, in the 1970's therapeutic care may have been coordinated through a type of individual treatment plan (e.g., Individual Habituation Plan) or some other team generated plan. Additionally, care providers were often on-site, which facilitated coordination and communication between providers and reduced the need for the individual with mental retardation to access community based health care services.

Other families during the 1940's and 50's opted to keep their children with disabilities at home, often sheltered from the community and without educational services. Many of these children, now adults, are becoming known to the mental health/mental retardation community only after the illness or death of caregivers force a need for residential placement.

In 1967 the deinstitutionalization movement shifted the primary focus away from placing persons with MR/DD into nursing homes and institutions and towards community placement, including group homes and family living (Ferguson, 1994). The passage of PL 94-142 in the mid 1970's expanded educational opportunities for individuals with MR/DD under the age of 21 (Education for All Handicapped Children, 1975). The focus of care shifted from care and housing to training. The philosophy of normalization promoted the concept that persons with MR/DD should experience a lifestyle similar to their same age peers, e.g., engaging in age appropriate activities (Nirje, 1969).

The focus of service delivery within the past decade has shifted from teaching the individual new skills to enhancing the individual's quality of life and increasing his/her participation in the local community. This paradigm shift has affected how services are delivered and the desired outcomes for service delivery. Instead of focusing on the development of skills and organizing the daily routine of an individual with MR/DD so that it resembled that of the typical person (Wolfensberger, 1972), services now focus on enhancing the individual's life satisfaction and increasing their participation in community activities (Dennis, Williams, Giancreco & Cloniger, 1993). More recently, the MR/DD community has focused on self-advocacy and empowerment. The national self-advocacy organization, Self Advocates Becoming Empowered, adopted the position that all people regardless of the severity of their disabilities should live in the community with the support they need (Cone, 1997). Further, they called for a closing of all institutions, private and public (Cone, 1997). Supporters of self-advocacy work to achieve human, civil and legal rights for persons with developmental disabilities through teaching members to speak out and advocate for themselves (Miller & Keys, 1996). Members also support accessible transportation, closing institutions, supported and competitive employment over sheltered employment, classroom inclusion, and choices in relationships and sexual expression (Miller & Keys, 1996).

Despite efforts to move people into the community, as late as 1992 there were still over 80,000 people with mental retardation living in large state run institutions (Ferguson, 1994). The majority of this group is diagnosed with severe and profound ranges of mental retardation (Cone, 1997).

CHALLENGES OF "AGING IN PLACE"

Aging in place in the community carries with it several challenges, especially for the elder adult with MR/DD, their families and service providers. Some of these challenges are faced by natural families who have been caring for their loved one for 50-60 years (Smith & Tobin, 1993). Farber (1959) described these families as "out of snyc" with their age peers whose children are grown and have left home. Families may be stuck in "perpetual parenting" (Jennings, 1987). An example of this is the need for families to find respite care or "babysitters" for the elder adult so that they may attend a social function. This long term caregiving may have significant effects on the primary caregiver, who is traditionally the mother (Smith & Tobin, 1993; Newbern & Hargett, 1992). Seltzer and Krauss (1989) noted that these mothers reported having a smaller social network than their same age peers who did not care for a child with a developmental disability. They also described their parenting role as a central part of their identity. Release of this caregiving role to another may be difficult due to the longevity and centrality of this role for the caregiver, the strong bond between parent and child and the mother's perception of the adult child's need for her support and care. These factors, along with cultural, religious, political or ethnic values regarding use of outside the family support systems may affect the family's use of respite care or other available support services or even the seeking of out-of-home placement for their child as they grow older (Smith & Tobin, 1993, Bromley & Blacher, 1989).

Janicki (1992) refers to families of adults with DD as the "two-generation elderly family" (p. 118). The parents' own energy and stamina begin to decline as they age, making the challenge of in-home care more difficult. The process of aging in the individual with MR/DD may result in decreased functioning and a need for increased support such as medical interventions, environmental modifications, and rehabilitative therapies. Parents report a decrease in the ability to provide care for their adult child as their own health problems increased (Engelhardt, Brubaker & Lutzer, 1988). Families need to consider long term planning such as changes in living arrangements, planning for changes in finances, guardianship, case management and recreation activities for their adult child. Heller and Factor (1991) interviewed families of adult children with MR/DD ranging in age from 21-70 years. They reported that families preferred placement in a family home (53%) to a residential program (4%) but that only 20% had made specific arrangements with a relative for a home placement, 7% had placed their relative on a waiting list for a residential program and 16% were beginning to investigate an alternative living arrangement.

Some of the challenges facing the elder adult with MR/DD result from the shift from institutional care to community living. These include: the limited number of community living homes available, the need for adequate training of staff to support these community homes, the coordination of therapeutic, medical and training services and the development of adequate programming to prepare elder adults with MR/DD for community integration.

Once a group home is established, staff training becomes an issue. Many facilities and agencies that operate group homes provide training for staff. However, in the United States the job of client caregiver is often an entry-level job, frequently filled by new high school graduates or college students. Staff turnover is generally high making continuity of care and program development difficult.

Another challenge is the coordination of medical and therapeutic services for elder adults with MR/DD living at home or in group homes. Unlike nursing homes and larger residential facilities that may employ medical and therapeutic staff, group homes and families rely on community services. Sometimes medical and therapeutic services are provided via contractual agreement. Service providers may have little opportunity to meet to coordinate services. Team decisions may be difficult to make in a timely manner which may result in delay of services such as program implementation or the procurement of wheelchairs or other assistive technology.

The following case study illustrates some of these challenges. Please note that in this and other case stories, the client's name has been changed to protect confidentiality.

Harry is 46 years old, non-verbal and diagnosed with autism and profound mental retardation. He came to live in a group home after forty years of living in a large state institution. He often engaged in self-injurious behavior when staff could not meet his need immediately. During visits from the OT, Harry was often seen standing near or leaning up against the refrigerator. Staff would attempt to predict Harry's needs, sometimes offering him a drink or snack or food. If it took too long for staff to guess his current need, Harry would engage in some negative behavior, such as head slapping or urinating.

Staff who worked with Harry on a consistent basis became quite good at guessing his needs. However, staff unfamiliar with Harry had great difficulty. The staff identified Harry's most pressing need as being able to let them know what he wants. The OT asked if picture charts or schedules had been used with Harry. They were not. The OT asked if a speech therapist had been working with Harry. There was not at this time, however, a speech therapist had previously been working with Harry to teach him sign language. The OT has brought in pictures and is evaluating Harry's potential to use these functionally to communicate. He is demonstrating limited success at this time. The OT believes staff commitment to this program is inconsistent.

This was an instance where therapists from two different disciplines responding to the needs of the client and staff generated two different solutions. The speech therapist had attempted to teach Harry sign language. The OT worked with Harry to use picture representation to tell staff his needs, thinking that pictures could be used to also develop a daily schedule to allow for a more predictable environment (something individuals with autism seem to respond well to). It would have been helpful if the two therapists had been able to communicate and work collaboratively to create one solution. This would help best meet the needs of the client, prevent therapists from implementing contradictory programs and not confuse the staff, client or client's family.

Also associated with the move to group homes is the need to prepare the adult with MR/DD before, during and after the transition. Persons with autism, for example, do not tend to respond well to changes and alterations in routine (Trevarthe, Aitken, Papoudi & Roboarts, 1996). A move from a family home or institution into a group home can be quite traumatic. Preparing the person through counseling and to the extent possible, site visits prior to the move would ease the transition into the new home. In one group for three adult men with autism and MR, staff and managers were very proactive in preparing clients prior to the move. They visited the clients in their current facility and brought them to "visit" the house before actually moving in. This was thought by many to ease the transition from the large institution to the smaller community home.

Other challenges face the elder adult with MR/DD and their service providers with regards to community integration. One is the idea of participating in retirement and leisure lifestyles. Elder adults with MR/DD may be working in competitive or supportive employment or in sheltered workshops or attending segregated day programs (Amado, Lakin & Menke, 1990). Several authors and researchers have developed models to facilitate integrated leisure services for the elder adult with MR/DD (Taylor, Biklen & Knoll, 1987; Carter & Foret, 1991; Keller, 1991; Zimpel, 1991). However, there remain significant barriers to integration. One is the belief that the needs of the elder adult are too significant and could not be met by generic services (Taylor et al., 1987; Roberto & Nelson, 1989). There also exist different perspectives as to the "best way" to meet those needs (Sison & Cotton, 1989). There appears to be a lack of available services (Riddick & Keller, 1991; Wilhite, Keller & Nicholson, 1991) and there are concerns regarding funding for these services (Tedrick, 1991).

Another issue is the quality and type of community health care services available to the elder adult with MR/DD. Several factors may impact medical care for the elder adult with MR/DD living in the community. One is the difficulty of determining the appropriate diagnosis and differentiating between the normal aging process and a disease state (Adlin, 1993). Several issues affect the health care team's ability to identify the appropriate diagnosis. These include, long term polypharmacy (Adlin, 1993), syndrome specific disabilities (Burt, Loveland, Yuan-Cho, Chuang, Lewis, & Cherry, 1995), the presence of chronic disease (Minihan & Dean, 1990), the physical aging process believed to be occurring earlier in some individuals with MR/DD (Seltzer & Seltzer, 1985), and the difficulty with differentiating between behavioral states and pain or discomfort (McGrath, Rosmus, Canfield, Campbell & Hennigar, 1998). Other barriers to medical care include the individual's inability to communicate a change in health status with the health care team, his/her inability to cooperate with some aspects of the medical examination (Ridenour & Norton, 1995) and decreased mobility in comparison with the general population (Beange et al., 1995). Another barrier to health care is the limited use of resources by caregivers who may assume an individual's behavior is related to his mental retardation or developmental disability and not indicative of a disease process (Ogunkua, 1998).

The concept of aging in place or remaining in the local community for as long as possible has impacted service delivery in major ways. Adults with MR/DD are moving from long term care facilities and nursing homes to smaller community based residence or remaining in family homes (Bradley & Allard, 1992; Barr, 1993). Agencies serving elder adults with MR/DD are moving toward greater use of community resources and informal support networks rather than institution based services (Anderson & Factor, 1993; Roberts & Sutton, 1993). Another issue is the availability of adequate funds to support service delivery to elder adults with MR/DD (Martinson & Stone, 1993). Funding issues have always and may always be a barrier to service delivery for individuals with MR/DD. As the population of elder adults with MR/DD continues to increase, new sources of funding will need to be created in order to meet their needs in the most appropriate way.

Sources of funding vary from state to state and within each state from county to county. Federal sources of funding include Medicaid (Title XIX of PL 74-271) and Medicare (Title XVIII of PL 74-271) programs, which support health-related services (Social Security Act of 1935, as amended, 1935). Other funding supports community living options such as the ICF/MR program (under Medicaid) and Home and Community-Based Care Services Waiver program (Social Security Act of 1935, as amended 1935). Other programs such as Technology-Related Assistance for Individuals with Disabilities Act of 1988, (1988) provide assistive technology to support community living options.

ROLE OF OCCUPATIONAL AND PHYSICAL THERAPISTS

Occupational and physical therapists play important roles in helping elder adults with MR/DD live meaningful lives within the community. While therapists cannot necessarily address each and every challenge facing the elder adult with MR/DD living in the community, therapists have unique expertise to offer to the elder adult client, their caregivers and service delivery team.

Occupational and physical therapists can offer support to the elder adult with MR/DD by working directly with the individual, through assessment and intervention, with his/her caregivers and/or health care team, and through assessing and modifying the environment in which the person will live or interact.

Therapists evaluate individual clients to determine their areas of strength and need. They develop individual intervention programs to prevent or remediate injuries related to developmental disabilities or aging, improve independence and to improve safety. Therapists work directly with the client to develop and learn specific skills, such as safe meal preparation and grooming, to increase independence in the home. Therapists should evaluate the client's community mobility requirements (shopping, doctor visits, community center) addressing the client's physical and cognitive needs to help the client participate in their community. Therapists should look at stressors in the client's life and environment and help the client develop appropriate coping skills.

To increase independence and safety, therapists may also need to train staff or family members to integrate intervention programs into the client's daily routines. Examples include training caregivers in functional transfers that are safe for both the client and the caregivers, recommending adaptive equipment for the home or developing an exercise program that caregivers can implement and monitor. Intervention programs designed to teach new skills should also be reviewed with staff or family to allow for consistency in presentation and ultimately provide the client a greater opportunity to learn the skill.

Therapists can also evaluate the environment and make recommendations for assistive technology, adaptive equipment and environmental modification, taking into account the client's current and potential needs. Recommendations may be related to ramps, stairs, furniture, bathroom safety, bed safety, or lighting. Consideration should be given to the client's current needs as well as future needs as the client's or family caregiver's age or as the client becomes more disabled. Therapists can also evaluate the environment outside the home and make recommendations for safe community integration such as sidewalks, traffic patterns, public transportation routes, proximity to stores and accessibility of community places.

Consideration must be given to the cost of the recommendations and the resources available to the caregivers. Consideration will also have to be given to the ability of the caregiver to implement the program based on his/her own physical and cognitive limitations and to the frequent staff turnover in some residential programs.

Occupational and physical therapists can work collaboratively with caregivers. This collaboration can take many forms. Early acknowledgement of the information the caregiver has of the elder adult client and involving them in the development of therapeutic programs may help the therapist develop a program with a greater chance of success. The therapist may work with caregivers early in the evaluation phase. Many elder adults with MR/DD are poor historians or are unable to give accurate information that is often part of the initial evaluation. Caregivers may recognize behavioral changes in the individual which may indicate pain such as changes in voice quality, eating or sleeping patterns, personality, facial expressions, activity level or other physiological changes (McGrath et al., 1998). Caregivers may also provide information as to what is expected of the client (vocational or home-making demands) or what the client enjoys doing (leisure pursuits). They may also give the therapist directives on the type of therapeutic program that is needed (e.g., emphasis on self-care vs. vocational preparedness). Therapists can provide training to group home staff, case managers, family members and other therapeutic and medical personnel who may not be familiar with the special needs of the client. This training can focus on specific client needs and programs as well as general issues of aging with a developmental disability. Therapists can provide specific training to staff responsible for implementing therapeutic programs. One time training is not sufficient. Ongoing staff training and program monitoring becomes a necessity.

Lastly, therapists are in a position to recommend appropriate programs and supports to promote the client's successful integration into the community, including participation in leisure and vocational activities. For example, a specific facility may be desirable for a client with orthopedic deformities because it does not involve a great deal of walking and there are no steps to enter the building. A specific job or leisure activity may be preferred for a client with cognitive limitations who requires specific set-up of materials and specific types of cues.

An example is Bob, a 47-year-old male diagnosed with mild mental retardation. Bob recently underwent surgery to stabilize his cervical spine. Post surgery he had to wear a cervical collar and ambulate using a rolling walker. Once the physician discharged the collar, Bob was able to return to work. The physical and occupational therapists toured

the work site. Together they generated the following recommendations: Bob would perform his job while sitting in a chair with arms and
without wheels that was at a functional height for the table. A raised
toilet seat with arms was ordered to make transfers easier and safer. A
platform was placed at the door of the van to allow Bob to transfer on
and off the bus safely. Bob also worked a shortened day to avoid
fatigue. These recommendations were implemented and Bob returned
to work with minimal cost to the employer and to Bob's residential
program.

Occupational and physical therapists working with local agencies
serving elder adults with MR/DD should be in close communication
with service coordinators and case managers. Innovative funding resources may be tapped in individual cases as the team explores specific issues and needs for the individual client. Examples include grant
funding for short-term projects, community fund raising, and collaboration with local business and industry to fund specific projects.

CONCLUSION

In many ways, the population of elder adults with MR/DD is new to
the community based health care profession. Current philosophy of
service support elder adults with MR/DD living, working and participating in local communities. This article discussed several of the key
issues affecting the elder adult with MR/DD aging in place in their local
community. This current perspective will create many opportunities for
occupational and physical therapists both now and in the future. As the
elder population continues to grow, more elder adults with MR/DD are
likely to require the services of an occupational and/or physical therapist. Therapists can offer direct and consultative service to help the
elder adult and his or her caregivers cope with the aging process while
maintaining the highest possible level of independence.

There are additional opportunities for occupational and physical
therapists who are interested in working specifically with the elder
adult with MR/DD and their caregivers. Specialized therapeutic skill
combined with a knowledge of gerontology and developmental disabilities will be required when working with the aging adult with
MR/DD. Therapists can also contribute to the limited knowledge base
regarding the aging process in the adult with MR/DD through clinical
research. Therapists can utilize their expertise to promote a healthier

life style, including the development of therapeutic exercise programs, assist in the participation of age appropriate day programs and community training to allow for more active participation in their communities. Therapists may be assuming roles as service coordinators to help families and caregivers attain the necessary services to assist the elder client in maintaining independence and aging successfully in community living opportunities.

REFERENCES

Adlin, M. (1993). Health care issues. In E. Sutton, A. Factor, B. Hawkins, T. Heller, & G. Seltzer (Eds.) *Older adults with developmental disabilities: Optimizing choice and change* (pp. 48-60). Baltimore: Paul H. Brookes, Pub. Co.

Amado, A. N., Lakin, K. C., & Menker, J. M. (1990). *Services for people with developmental disabilities.* Minneapolis, MN: University of Minnesota, Center for Residential and Community Services.

Anderson, D. J. (1993). Health issues. In E. Sutton, A. Factor, B. Hawkins, T. Heller, & G. Seltzer (Eds.) *Older adults with developmental disabilities: Optimizing choice and change* (pp. 29-48). Baltimore: Paul H. Brookes, Pub. Co.

Anderson, D. J. & Factor, A. (1993, Spring). Person-centered planning in case Coordination. *Impact, 6*(1), 4-5.

Barr, O. (1993) Community homes: Institutions in waiting? *Nursing Standard 7*(41), 34-37.

Beange, H., McElduff, A., & Baker, W. (1995). Medical disorders of adults with mental retardation: A population study. *American Journal on Mental Retardation, 99*(6), 595-604.

Bonder B. & Wagner, M. (1994). *Functional performance in older adults.* Philadelphia: F. A. Davis.

Bradley, V. & Allard, M. A. (1992). The dynamics of change in residential services for people with developmental disabilities. In J. W. Jacobson, S. N. Burchard & P. J. Carling (Eds.) *Community Living for People with Developmental and Psychiatric Disabilities* (pp. 284-302). Baltimore: Johns Hopkins University Press.

Burt, D., Loveland, K. Yuan-Cho, C. Chuang, A., Lewis, K. & Cherry, L. (1995). Aging in adults with Down Syndrome: Report from a longitudinal study. *American Journal of Mental Retardation, 100*(3), 262-270.

Bromley, B. & Blacher, J. (1989). Factors delaying out-of-home placement of children with severe handicaps. *American Journal of Mental Retardation, 94*, 284-291.

Carter, M. & Foret, C. (1991). Therapeutic recreation–programming for older adults with developmental disabilities. *Activities with Developmentally Disabled Elderly and Older Adults. 16*(1/2), 35-51.

Chicoine, B. & McGuire, D. (1997). Longevity of a woman with Down Syndrome: A case study. *Mental Retardation, 35*(5), 477-479.

Cone, A. (1997). The beat goes on: Lessons learned from the rhythms of the self-advocacy movement. *Mental Retardation, 35*(2), 144-145.

Connolly, B. H. (1998). General effects of aging on persons with developmental disabilities. *Topics in Geriatric Rehabilitation, 13*(3), 1-18.

Dennis, R. E., Williams, W., Giancreco, M. F. & Cloninger, C. J. (1993). Quality of life as context for planning and evaluation for services for people with disabilities. *Exceptional Children, 59*(6), 499-512.

DiGiovanni, L. (1978). The elderly retarded: A little known group. *Gerontologist, 18*(3), 262-266.

Edgerton, R., B., Gaston, M. A., Kelly, H. & Ward, T. W. (1994). Health care for aging people with mental retardation. *Mental Retardation, 32*(2) 146-150.

Education for All Handicapped Children, PL 94-142, U.S. Congress, Senate, 94th Congress, First Session (1975).

Engelhardt, J., Brubaker, T. & Lutzer, V. (1988). Older caregivers of adults with mental retardation: Service utilization. *Mental Retardation, 26,* 191-195.

Farber, B. (1959). *Effects of a severely mentally retarded child on family integration.* Monographs of the Society for Research in Child Development (Serial No. 17).

Ferguson, P. (1994). *Abandoned to their fate.* Philadelphia: Temple University Press.

Foelker, G. A., & Luke, E. A. (1989). Mental health issues for the aging mentally retarded population. *Journal of Applied Gerontology, 8,* 242-250.

Heller, T. & Factor., A. (1991). Permanency planning for adults with mental retardation living with family caregivers. *American Journal on Mental Retardation, 96,* 163-176.

Herge, E. A. & Campbell, J. E. (1999). Older adults with mental retardation: Challenges and opportunities. *OT Practice, 4*(5),16-21.

Janicki, M. (1992). Lifelong disability and aging. In L. Rowitz (Ed.), *Mental retardation in the year 2000* (pp.115-127). New York: Springer-Verlag.

Jennings, J. (1987). Elderly parents as caregivers for their adult dependent children. *Social Work, 32,* 430-433.

Kapell, D., Nightingale, B., Rodriquez, A., Lee, J. H., Zigman, W. B., & Schupf, N. (1998). Prevalence of chronic medical conditions in adults with mental retardation: Comparison with the general population. *Mental Retardation, 36*(4), 269-279.

Keller, M. J. (1991). Creating a recreation integration process among older adults with mental retardation. *Educational Gerontology, 17,* 275-288.

Martinson, M.C. & Stone, J. A. (1993). Federal legislation and long-term funding streams that support community living options. In E. Sutton, A. Factor, B. Hawkins, T. Heller, & G. Seltzer (Eds.) *Older adults with developmental disabilities: Optimizing choice and change* (pp.199-221). Baltimore: Paul H. Brookes, Pub. Co.

McGrath, P., Rosmus, C., Canfield, C., Campbell, M.A., & Henningar, A. (1998). Behaviours caregivers use to determine pain in non-verbal, cognitively impaired individuals. *Developmental Medicine & Child Neurology, 40*(5), 340-343.

Miller, A. B. & Keys, K. B. (1996). Awareness, action, and collaboration: How the self-advocacy movement is empowering for persons with developmental disabilities. *Mental Retardation, 34*(5), 312-319.

Minnihan, P. H. & Dean, D. H. (1990). Meeting the needs for health services of persons with mental retardation living in the community. *American Journal of Public Health, 80*(9), 1043-1048.

Nirje, B. (1969). The normalization principle. In R. B. Kiegel (Ed.). *Changing patterns in residential services for the mentally retarded.* Washington: President's Committee on Mental Retardation.

Newbern, V. & Hargett, M. (1992). A gerontological nursing issue: The aged developmentally disabled/mentally retarded. *Holistic Nursing Practice, 7*(1), 70-77.

Ogunkua, B. (1998). *Growing old in a new age: Medical health aspects of aging in people with developmental disabilities.* Paper presented at the meeting of Montgomery County MH/MR Providers, Conshohocken, PA.

Riddick, C. C. & Keller, M. J. (1991). Developing recreation services to assist elders who are developmentally disabled. *Activities with Developmentally Disabled Elderly and Older Adults, 16*(1/2), 19-33.

Ridenour, N. & Norton, D. (1995). Community-based persons with mental retardation: Opportunities for health promotion. *Nurse Practitioner Forum, 61*(1), 19-23.

Roberto, K. & Nelson, R. E. (1989). The developmentally disabled elderly: Concerns of service providers. *Journal of Applied Gerontology, 8,* 175-182.

Roberts, R. S. & Sutton, E. (1993, Spring). Integrated leisure options: The peer companion model. *Impact, 6*(1), 13.

Rojahn, J., Warren, V. J. & Ohringer, S. (1994). A comparison of assessment methods for depression in mental retardation. *Journal of Autism and Developmental Disorders, 24*(3), 305-313.

Rowles, G. D. (1993). Evolving images of place in aging and "aging in place." *Generations, 17*(2), 65-71.

Seltzer, M. M. & Seltzer, G. B. (1985). The elderly mentally retarded: A group in need of service. *Journal of Gerontological Social Work, 8,* 99-119.

Seltzer, M. & Krauss, M. (1989). Aging parents with adult mentally retarded children: Family risk factors and sources of support. *American Journal of Mental Retardation, 94,* 303-312.

Sison, G. F. P. & Cotton, P. D. (1989). The elderly mentally retarded person: Current perspectives and future directions. *Journal of Applied Gerontology, 8*(2), 151-167.

Smith, G. C. & Tobin, S. S. (1993). Practice with older parents of developmentally disabled adults. *Clinical Gerontolgoist, 14*(1), 59-77.

Social Security Act of 1935 as Amended, PL 74-271. US Congress, Senate, 74th Congress, First Session. (1935).

Taylor, S. J., Biklen, D. & Knoll, J. (1987). *Community integration for people with severe disabilities.* New York: Teachers College Press.

Technology-Related Assistance for Individuals with Disabilities Act of 1988, PL 100-407, US Congress, Senate, 100th Congress, Second Session (1988).

Tedrick, T. (1991). Aging, developmental disabilities and leisure: Policy and service delivery issues. *Activities with Developmentally Disabled Elderly and Older Adults, 16*(1/2), 141-152.

Trevarthe, C., Aitken, K., Papoudi, D., & Roboarts, J. (1996). *Children with autism: Diagnoses and interventions to meet their needs.* London: Jessica Kingsley Publishers.

Wilhite, B., Keller, M. J. & Nicholson, L. (1991). Integrating older persons with developmental disabilities into community recreation: Theory to practice. *Activities with Developmentally Disabled Elderly and Older Adults. 16*(1/2), 111-129.

Wolfensberger, W. (1972). *Normalization: The principle of normalization in human services.* Toronto: Leonard Crainford.

Wolfensberger, W. (1991). Reflections on a lifetime in human services and mental retardation. *Mental Retardation, 29*(1), 1-15.

Zimpel, B. (1991). Sharing activities-The Oneida County A. R. C. Cornhill Senior Center project, *Activities with Developmentally Disabled Elderly and Older Adults, 16*(1/2), 131-139.

Aging and Developmental Disability Information Resources

Joy Hammel, PhD, OTR/L, FAOTA

Following are useful sources of information on aging and developmental disability policy, services, education and research. Many have information clearinghouses from which you can order publications, monographs, current reports, training guides and resource listings. Their websites link you to many other related sites, organizations, databases, conferences and products.

Administration on Developmental Disabilities (ADD)

U.S. Department of Health and Human Services
Mail Stop: HHH 300-F, 370 L'Enfant Promenade, S.W.
Washington, DC 20447
WWW: *http://www.acf.dhhs.gov/programs/add/*

The Administration on Developmental Disabilities (ADD) is the federal agency that administers four national programs: State Developmental Disabilities Councils (DDCs), Protection and Advocacy Programs (P&As), University Affiliated Programs (UAPs), and Projects of National Significance (PNS). The website contains descriptions of each program and links to state and local organizations throughout the country that have a wealth of current information on aging and developmental disability.

Joy Hammel is Assistant Professor, Occupational Therapy Department, University of Illinois at Chicago, 1919 West Taylor Street, Room 311, Chicago, IL 60612 (E-mail: hammel@uic.edu).

[Haworth co-indexing entry note]: "Aging and Developmental Disability Information Resources." Hammel, Joy. Co-published simultaneously in *Physical & Occupational Therapy in Geriatrics* (The Haworth Press, Inc.) Vol. 18, No. 1, 2000, pp. 91-94; and: *Aging and Developmental Disability: Current Research, Programming, and Practice Implications* (ed: Joy Hammel, and Susan M. Nochajski) The Haworth Press, Inc., 2000, pp. 91-94. Single or multiple copies of this article are available for a fee from The Haworth Document Delivery Service [1-800-342-9678, 9:00 a.m. - 5:00 p.m. (EST). E-mail address: getinfo@haworthpressinc.com].

National Organizations That Provide Information Resources (Publications, Conferences, Research Reports, Local Chapters, Websites and Links to Our Many Sources of Information on Aging and Developmental Disability)

American Association on Mental Retardation (AAMR)
444 North Capitol Street, NW, Suite 846, Washington, DC 20001-1512
(202) 387-1968 or (800) 424-3688; Fax: (202) 387-2193
WWW: *http://www.aamr.org*

The Arc (formally known as the Association for Retarded Citizens)
1010 Wayne Ave., Suite 650, Silver Spring, MD 20910
(301) 565-3842
WWW: *http://www.thearc.org/*

(The Arc and the Rehabilitation Research and Training Center on Aging with Mental Retardation have just released a new 8-page fact sheet entitled, *"Aging with Developmental Disabilities: Women's Health Issues."* The fact sheet is available at no cost in PDF and HTML formats at: *http://TheArc.org/faqs/whealthindx.html*)

United Cerebral Palsy (UCP)
1660 L St., NW, Suite 700, Washington, DC 20036-5603
(800) USA-5-UCP or (202) 776-0406; TTY: (202) 973-7197;
Fax: (202) 776-0414
E-mail: *ucpnatl@ucpa.org*
WWW: *http://www.ucpa.org/*

TASH (previously known as The Association for Persons with Severe Handicaps)
29 W. Susquehanna Avenue, Suite 210, Baltimore, MD 21204
(410) 828-8274; Fax (410) 828-6706
WWW: *http://www.tash.org/misc/index.htm*

National Institute on Disability and Rehabilitation Research (NIDRR) Centers

Federally funded centers that conduct research, provide training and technical assistance, and develop and test new programs and products in areas related to aging and developmental disability (see: *http://www.ed.gov/offices/OSERS/NIDRR/* for complete listings of all NIDRR-funded projects and programs).

Rehabilitation Research and Training Center on Aging with Mental Retardation
University of Illinois-Chicago
Department of Disability and Human Development
1640 West Roosevelt Road, Chicago, IL 60608-6904
(312) 413-1520; Fax: (312) 996-6942; TDD: (312) 413-0453
WWW: *http://www.uic.edu/orgs/rrtcamr/*

The RRTCAMR's Clearinghouse on Aging and Developmental Disabilities disseminates research findings, curricula, manuals, fact sheets, the A/DDvantage newsletter, and other publications. The Clearinghouse also contains a computerized database of over 2,000 reprints, bibliographies, manuals, and monographs. The Center also sponsors the Electronic Discussion List (Listserv) on DD/Aging Women's Health: To subscribe to the forum, send an e-mail message to Listserv@listserv.uic.edu, and type: *Subscribe WomHlthAging-DD <YourFirstName> <YourLastName>*

Rehabilitation Research and Training Center on Aging with a Disability
Rancho Los Amigos Medical Center
Los Amigos Research & Education Institute, Inc. (LAREI)
7601 East Imperial Highway, 800 West Annex, Downey, CA 90242
Voice: (562) 401-7402; Fax: (562) 401-7011; TDD: (562) 803-4533
WWW: *http://www.usc.edu/dept/gero/RRTConAging/index.html*

Rehabilitation Engineering and Research Center on Aging
State University of New York at Buffalo
Center for Assistive Technology
515 Kimball Tower, Buffalo, NY 14214-3079
Voice/Text Telephone: (800) 628-2281; Fax: (716) 829-3217
WWW: *http://wings.buffalo.edu/ot/cat/rerca.htm*

Websites with Links to Related Resources, Research, Products and Publications

- National Information Center on Developmental Disabilities (NICDD):
  http://www.acf.dhhs.gov/programs/add/NICDD/nicdd.htm
- Comprehensive Disability Internet Index:
  http://www.igc.apc.org/pwd/index.html

- National Rehabilitation Information Center (NARIC):
  http://www.naric.com/naric/
- National Center for the Dissemination of Disability Research:
  http://www.ncddr.org/
- Self Advocates Becoming Empowered (SABE):
  http://www.sabeusa.org/
- Research Homepage for Older Women with Disabilities:
  http://www.uic.edu/~lisab/homepage.htm
- Center for Research on Women with Disabilities:
  http://www.bcm.tmc.edu/crowd/baylor2.html
- RESNA: Rehabilitation Engineering and Assistive Technology Society of North America:
  http://www.resna.org/
- Technical Assistance Projects (TAPs):
  http://www.resna.org/taproject/index.html
- Closing the Gap: Computer Technology in Special Education and Rehabilitation:
  http://www.closingthegap.com/
- Rehab Central:
  http://www.rehabcentral.com/index.cfm
- Family Village:
  http://www.familyvillage.wisc.edu/index.htmlx
- The Boulevard:
  http://www.blvd.com/

Index

Numbers followed by a "t" indicate a table.